DR. HERMIONE MENDEZ

DIABETIC RENAL DIET

COOKBOOK FOR SENIORS

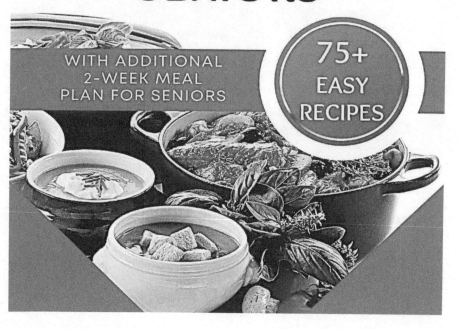

WITH ADDITIONAL
2-WEEK MEAL
PLAN FOR SENIORS

75+
EASY
RECIPES

DIABETIC RENAL

DIET COOKBOOK

FOR SENIORS

The Complete Seniors' Low-Salt, Low-Sugar, Low-Potassium, and Low-Phosphorus Diet To Reversing Diabetes and Kidney Disease With Easy Cooking

Dr. Hermione Mendez

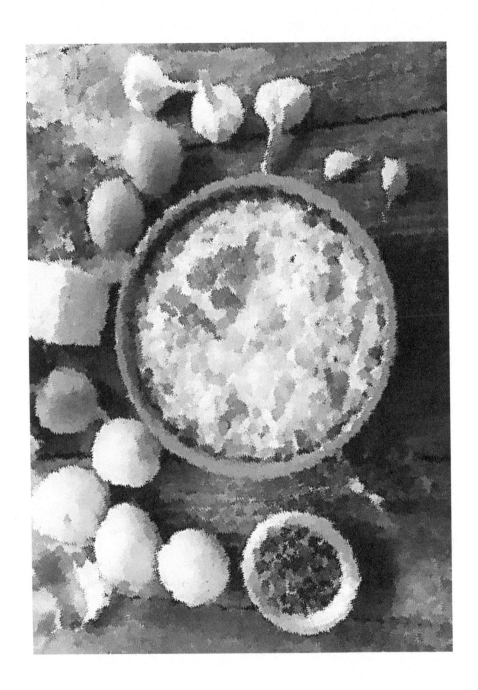

TABLE OF CONTENTS

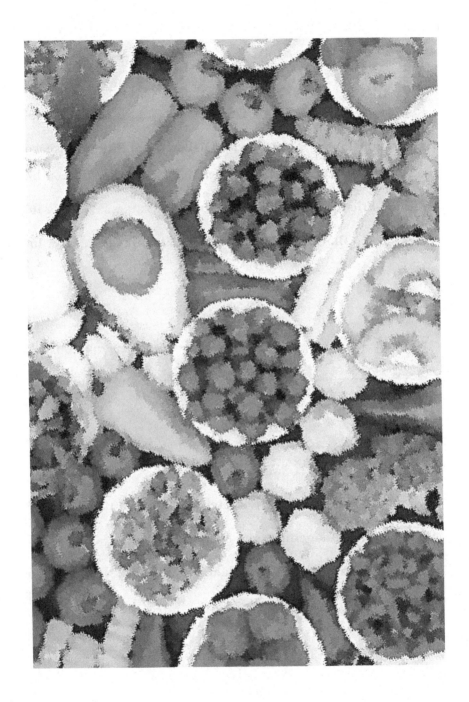

8

INTRODUCTION

Welcome to the Diabetic Renal Diet Cookbook for Seniors!

This cookbook is specially designed to provide guidance and support for seniors who are managing diabetes and kidney disease. I understand the unique challenges and dietary considerations that come with these health conditions, and my goal is to help you embrace a delicious and fulfilling lifestyle while prioritizing your well-being.

As we age, our bodies undergo changes, and it becomes increasingly important to maintain a healthy diet to support our overall health. For seniors with diabetes and kidney disease, this means paying careful attention to what we eat and ensuring that our meals are both nourishing and enjoyable.

Managing diabetes and kidney disease simultaneously requires a delicate balance of monitoring blood glucose levels, limiting sodium intake, and controlling the consumption of certain nutrients like potassium and phosphorus. It can feel overwhelming at times, but with the right knowledge and guidance, it is possible to create a sustainable and enjoyable eating plan.

In this cookbook, I have compiled a wide range of recipes that are tailored to meet the nutritional needs of seniors with diabetes and kidney disease. Each recipe is carefully crafted to strike a balance between taste, health, and ease of preparation. We have taken great care to consider the specific dietary restrictions associated with these conditions, while still ensuring that every dish is packed with flavor and variety.

Furthermore, this cookbook is not just about providing recipes. I aim to empower you with knowledge and practical tips to help you navigate your dietary journey with confidence. Within these pages, you will find information on understanding diabetes and kidney health, meal planning strategies, portion control techniques, and ingredient substitutions to meet your dietary requirements.

It's time to embrace a renewed sense of well-being and savor the joys of delicious, kidney-friendly meals. Let this cookbook be your guide as you embark on a culinary adventure that prioritizes your health and happiness.

Here's to good health and delightful dining experiences!

Sincerely,

Dr. Hermione Mendez.

UNDERSTANDING DIABETES AND RENAL HEALTH

DIABETES AND KIDNEY DISEASE: A COMPLEX RELATIONSHIP

Diabetes and kidney disease often go hand in hand. Diabetes is a chronic metabolic disorder characterized by high blood glucose levels resulting from insulin resistance or insufficient insulin production. When diabetes is not well-managed, it can lead to complications such as kidney disease, also known as diabetic nephropathy.

The kidneys play a crucial role in filtering waste products and excess fluids from the blood, maintaining fluid balance, and regulating blood pressure. However, prolonged high blood glucose levels and uncontrolled diabetes can damage the small blood vessels in the kidneys, impairing their ability to function properly. This damage can progress over time, leading to chronic kidney disease (CKD) or even end-stage renal disease (ESRD), where dialysis or kidney transplantation becomes necessary.

11

MANAGING DIABETES AND RENAL HEALTH AS A SENIOR:

Seniors face unique challenges in managing both diabetes and renal health. Age-related factors, such as decreased kidney function and potential complications from long-term diabetes, require careful attention and specialized dietary modifications. Additionally, seniors may be more prone to other health conditions, making the management of diabetes and renal health even more critical.

- Regular Monitoring: Seniors should monitor their blood glucose levels, kidney function, and blood pressure regularly. Regular check-ups and consultations with healthcare professionals are essential for managing these conditions effectively.

- Medication Management: Seniors with diabetes and kidney disease may require multiple medications to control their blood glucose levels, blood pressure, and other related factors. It is crucial to adhere to medication schedules and discuss any concerns or side effects with healthcare providers.

- Balanced Diabetic Renal Diet: Following a well-planned diabetic renal diet is vital for seniors. This diet focuses on managing blood glucose levels, reducing sodium intake, and controlling potassium and phosphorus levels. It emphasizes nutrient-dense, low-glycemic index foods while limiting processed foods, added sugars, and high-sodium ingredients.

TIPS FOR FOLLOWING A DIABETIC RENAL DIET:

- Carbohydrate Monitoring: Seniors should monitor their carbohydrate intake to manage blood glucose levels effectively. Choosing complex carbohydrates with a low glycemic index, such as whole grains, legumes, and non-starchy vegetables, can help stabilize blood sugar levels.

- Sodium Restriction: Reducing sodium intake is crucial for managing blood pressure and preventing fluid retention in individuals with kidney disease. Seniors should limit their consumption of processed foods, canned goods, and high-sodium condiments while opting for fresh herbs, spices, and homemade meals.

- Potassium and Phosphorus Control: Seniors with kidney disease often need to limit their potassium and phosphorus intake. Choosing low-potassium fruits and vegetables and properly leaching high-potassium vegetables can help manage potassium levels. Additionally, avoiding high-phosphorus foods like processed meats, dairy products, and certain grains is essential.

- Fluid Management: Seniors with kidney disease may require fluid restrictions, depending on their individual circumstances. Consulting with healthcare professionals to determine an appropriate fluid intake level is crucial to maintain fluid balance and prevent complications.

Understanding the relationship between diabetes and renal health is vital for seniors looking to manage their conditions effectively.

By following a diabetic renal diet tailored to their individual needs, seniors can take proactive steps to support their overall well-being. Being mindful of carbohydrate intake, controlling sodium and protein levels, and incorporating kidney-friendly foods are key strategies for maintaining optimal health. Regular consultation with healthcare professionals and adherence to a well-rounded management plan can help seniors thrive while managing diabetes and kidney disease.

CHAPTER 1: PLANNING A DIABETIC RENAL DIET FOR SENIORS

MEAL PLANNING BASICS

Planning a balanced and nutritious diet is essential for seniors managing diabetes and renal health. A diabetic renal meal plan focuses on controlling blood sugar levels while also considering the dietary restrictions associated with kidney disease. By following a well-designed meal plan, seniors can effectively manage their conditions and improve overall well-being.

CREATING A BALANCED DIABETIC RENAL MEAL PLAN

A balanced diabetic renal meal plan incorporates a variety of nutrient-dense foods that provide essential vitamins, minerals, and fiber while controlling blood glucose levels and minimizing stress on the kidneys. It is important to consult with a healthcare professional or a registered dietitian to tailor the meal plan to individual needs. Here are some key components to consider when creating a balanced meal plan:

- Carbohydrates: Selecting the right types and amounts of carbohydrates is crucial for blood sugar management. Focus on complex carbohydrates with a low glycemic index, such as whole grains, legumes, and non-starchy vegetables. These foods provide a steady release of glucose into the bloodstream and help maintain stable blood sugar levels.

- Protein: Opt for lean sources of protein, such as skinless poultry, fish, tofu, and legumes. Adequate protein intake is essential for tissue repair and maintenance, but excessive protein consumption can put strain on the kidneys. Consult with a healthcare professional to determine the appropriate protein intake based on individual needs and kidney function.

- Fats: Include healthy fats in the diet, such as monounsaturated fats found in olive oil, avocados, and nuts. These fats support heart health and provide a feeling of satiety. However, it is important to moderate fat intake to maintain a healthy weight, as excess weight can contribute to insulin resistance and kidney complications.

- Fiber: Incorporate high-fiber foods, including fruits, vegetables, whole grains, and legumes, into the meal plan. Fiber helps regulate blood sugar levels, promotes healthy digestion, and aids in maintaining a healthy weight. Aim for a variety of fiber-rich foods to maximize nutritional benefits.

- Hydration: Stay hydrated by drinking adequate fluids throughout the day. Water is the best choice, but herbal teas, infused water, and low-sugar beverages can also contribute to hydration. Adequate hydration supports kidney function and helps prevent complications related to diabetes and kidney disease.

PORTION CONTROL AND MONITORING CARBOHYDRATE INTAKE

Portion control plays a vital role in managing blood sugar levels and promoting overall health for seniors with diabetes and kidney disease. Measuring and monitoring portion sizes can help maintain stable blood glucose levels and prevent excessive calorie intake, which can lead to weight gain and increased strain on the kidneys. Consider the following strategies:

- Use measuring tools: Use measuring cups, spoons, and a food scale to accurately measure portion sizes. This practice helps to avoid overeating and provides a better understanding of the nutritional content of each meal.

- Read food labels: Pay attention to serving sizes listed on food labels to determine the appropriate portion size for a particular food item. Be mindful of carbohydrate content, as carbohydrates have the most significant impact on blood sugar levels.

- Balanced plate method: Divide your plate into sections to ensure a balanced meal. Fill half of the plate with non-starchy vegetables, one-fourth with lean protein, and one-fourth with whole grains or starchy vegetables. This method helps control portion sizes and encourages a variety of nutrient-rich foods.

- Glycemic index: Consider the glycemic index (GI) of carbohydrates. Foods with a high GI cause a more rapid increase in blood sugar levels. Choose foods with a low or moderate GI to help control blood glucose levels more effectively.

INCORPORATING LOW-SUGAR, LOW-SODIUM, LOW-POTASSIUM, AND LOW-PHOSPHORUS FOODS

For seniors managing both diabetes and kidney disease, it is crucial to incorporate foods that are low in sugar, sodium, potassium, and phosphorus. These dietary considerations help maintain stable blood glucose levels, reduce the risk of cardiovascular complications, and alleviate stress on the kidneys. Here are some suggestions for each category:

LOW-SUGAR FOODS:

- Choose fresh fruits with a low glycemic index, such as berries, cherries, and apples.
- Opt for sugar-free or naturally sweetened alternatives, such as stevia or monk fruit, instead of regular table sugar.
- Limit the consumption of sugary beverages, processed snacks, and desserts that can cause blood sugar spikes.

LOW-SODIUM FOODS:

- Use herbs and spices to season meals instead of salt. Experiment with flavors like garlic, ginger, cumin, and lemon juice.
- Select fresh or frozen vegetables without added salt. If using canned vegetables, rinse them under water to reduce sodium content.
- Choose low-sodium or salt-free versions of condiments, sauces, and canned goods.

LOW-POTASSIUM FOODS:

- Include low-potassium fruits such as apples, berries, and grapes in the diet.
- Opt for vegetables with lower potassium content, such as green beans, cauliflower, and bell peppers.
- Limit high-potassium foods like bananas, oranges, tomatoes, potatoes, and spinach, as they can raise potassium levels in the blood.

LOW-PHOSPHORUS FOODS:

- Choose lean protein sources with lower phosphorus content, such as chicken breast, fish, and tofu.
- Consume grains and cereals with lower phosphorus levels, like rice, corn, and oats.
- Limit high-phosphorus foods, including dairy products, nuts, seeds, and processed foods.

It is essential to consult with a healthcare professional or a registered dietitian to determine the appropriate restrictions and allowances for each individual's specific condition and stage of kidney disease.

By following a well-planned diabetic renal meal plan that incorporates portion control, monitoring carbohydrate intake, and selecting low-sugar, low-sodium, low-potassium, and low-phosphorus foods, seniors can effectively manage their diabetes and renal health.

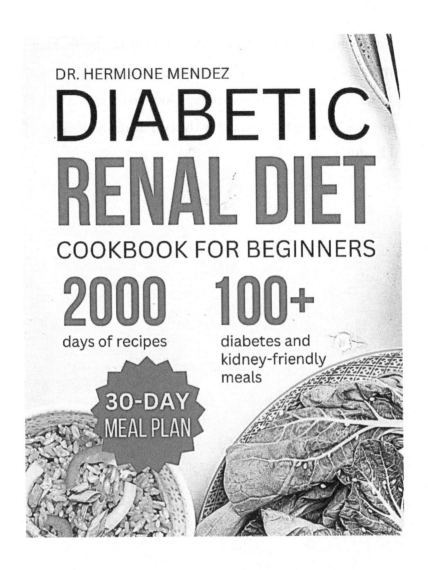

GET ON AMAZON TODAY!

CHAPTER 2: DIABETIC RENAL BREAKFASTS

SCRUMPTIOUS OATMEAL VARIATIONS:

BLUEBERRY ALMOND OATMEAL

Time: 15 minutes

Servings: 2

Ingredients:

- 1 cup old-fashioned oats
- 2 cups water
- 1/2 cup fresh or frozen blueberries
- 2 tablespoons unsalted almond butter
- 2 tablespoons chopped almonds
- Cinnamon (optional)

Directions:

- In a medium saucepan, bring the water to a boil.

- Add the oats and reduce the heat to low. Cook for about 5 minutes, stirring occasionally, until the oats are tender and the mixture thickens.
- Stir in the blueberries and continue cooking for an additional 2 minutes, until the berries are heated through.
- Remove the oatmeal from the heat and stir in the almond butter until well combined.
- Divide the oatmeal into two bowls and sprinkle with chopped almonds. Add a dash of cinnamon, if desired.
- Serve warm and enjoy!

Nutritional Information:

- Calories: 250
- Carbohydrates: 33g
- Protein: 9g
- Fat: 10g
- Sodium: 5mg
- Potassium: 180mg
- Phosphorus: 150mg

CINNAMON APPLE OATMEAL

Time: 15 minutes

Servings: 2

Ingredients:

- 1 cup old-fashioned oats
- 2 cups water
- 1 small apple, peeled and diced
- 1/2 teaspoon ground cinnamon
- 2 tablespoons chopped walnuts
- Unsweetened almond milk (optional, for serving)

Directions:

- In a medium saucepan, bring the water to a boil.
- Add the oats and reduce the heat to low. Cook for about 5 minutes, stirring occasionally, until the oats are tender and the mixture thickens.
- Stir in the diced apple and ground cinnamon. Continue cooking for an additional 2-3 minutes, until the apple is soft.
- Remove the oatmeal from the heat and divide it into two bowls.
- Sprinkle chopped walnuts on top of each bowl.
- If desired, drizzle a small amount of unsweetened almond milk over the oatmeal before serving.
- Enjoy while warm!

Nutritional Information:

- Calories: 230
- Carbohydrates: 34g
- Protein: 6g
- Fat: 8g
- Sodium: 5mg
- Potassium: 180mg
- Phosphorus: 150mg

COCONUT AND PINEAPPLE OATMEAL

Time: 15 minutes

Servings: 2

Ingredients:

- 1 cup old-fashioned oats
- 2 cups water
- 1/4 cup unsweetened shredded coconut
- 1/2 cup diced pineapple (fresh or canned in juice)
- 2 tablespoons chopped macadamia nuts
- Unsweetened coconut milk (optional, for serving)

Directions:

- In a medium saucepan, bring the water to a boil.

- Add the oats and reduce the heat to low. Cook for about 5 minutes, stirring occasionally, until the oats are tender and the mixture thickens.
- Stir in the shredded coconut and diced pineapple. Cook for an additional 2 minutes, until the pineapple is heated through.
- Remove the oatmeal from the heat and divide it into two bowls.
- Sprinkle chopped macadamia nuts on top of each bowl.
- If desired, drizzle a small amount of unsweetened coconut milk over the oatmeal before serving.
- Enjoy while warm!

Nutritional Information:

- Calories: 260
- Carbohydrates: 36g
- Protein: 6g
- Fat: 11g
- Sodium: 5mg
- Potassium: 200mg
- Phosphorus: 150mg

PEANUT BUTTER BANANA OATMEAL

Time: 15 minutes

Servings: 2

Ingredients:

- 1 cup old-fashioned oats
- 2 cups water
- 2 tablespoons natural peanut butter
- 1 medium banana, sliced
- 1 tablespoon chopped peanuts (unsalted)
- Cinnamon (optional)

Directions:

- In a medium saucepan, bring the water to a boil.
- Add the oats and reduce the heat to low. Cook for about 5 minutes, stirring occasionally, until the oats are tender and the mixture thickens.
- Stir in the peanut butter until it is fully incorporated into the oatmeal.
- Remove the oatmeal from the heat and divide it into two bowls.
- Top each bowl with sliced banana and chopped peanuts.
- Add a sprinkle of cinnamon, if desired.
- Serve warm and enjoy!

Nutritional Information:

- Calories: 310

- Carbohydrates: 40g

- Protein: 11g

- Fat: 13g

- Sodium: 5mg

- Potassium: 290mg

- Phosphorus: 200mg

MAPLE PECAN OATMEAL

Time: 15 minutes

Servings: 2

Ingredients:

- 1 cup old-fashioned oats

- 2 cups water

- 2 tablespoons chopped pecans

- 2 teaspoons pure maple syrup

- 1/2 teaspoon vanilla extract

- Unsweetened almond milk (optional, for serving)

Directions:

- In a medium saucepan, bring the water to a boil.

- Add the oats and reduce the heat to low. Cook for about 5 minutes, stirring occasionally, until the oats are tender and the mixture thickens.
- Stir in the chopped pecans, maple syrup, and vanilla extract. Cook for an additional 2 minutes, until the pecans are fragrant.
- Remove the oatmeal from the heat and divide it into two bowls.
- If desired, drizzle a small amount of unsweetened almond milk over the oatmeal before serving.
- Enjoy while warm!

Nutritional Information:

- Calories: 280
- Carbohydrates: 39g
- Protein: 7g
- Fat: 11g
- Sodium: 5mg
- Potassium: 160mg
- Phosphorus: 120mg

FLAVORFUL EGG DISHES WITH LOW SODIUM OPTIONS:

VEGGIE-PACKED EGG WHITE OMELET

Time: 15 minutes

Servings: 1

Ingredients:

- 4 egg whites
- 1/4 cup diced bell peppers
- 1/4 cup diced onions
- 1/4 cup diced tomatoes
- 1/4 cup chopped spinach
- 2 tablespoons crumbled feta cheese
- Cooking spray
- Salt and pepper to taste

Directions:

- In a bowl, whisk the egg whites until frothy. Season with salt and pepper.
- Heat a non-stick skillet over medium heat and coat with cooking spray.
- Add the bell peppers, onions, and tomatoes to the skillet and sauté until softened.
- Add the chopped spinach to the skillet and cook until wilted.
- Pour the whisked egg whites over the vegetables in the skillet.
- Sprinkle the crumbled feta cheese evenly over the egg whites.

- Cook for a few minutes until the edges are set, then carefully fold the omelet in half.
- Continue cooking until the omelet is fully set and lightly golden.
- Slide the omelet onto a plate and serve hot.

Nutritional Information:

- Calories: 150
- Protein: 26g
- Fat: 4g
- Carbohydrates: 7g
- Fiber: 2g
- Sodium: 250mg
- Potassium: 300mg
- Phosphorus: 100mg

SPINACH AND FETA SCRAMBLED EGGS

Time: 10 minutes

Servings: 1

Ingredients:

- 2 whole eggs
- 1/2 cup chopped spinach

- 1 tablespoon crumbled feta cheese
- Cooking spray
- Salt and pepper to taste

Directions:

- In a bowl, whisk the eggs until well beaten. Season with salt and pepper.
- Heat a non-stick skillet over medium heat and coat with cooking spray.
- Add the chopped spinach to the skillet and sauté until wilted.
- Pour the beaten eggs over the spinach in the skillet.
- Sprinkle the crumbled feta cheese evenly over the eggs.
- Stir gently and continuously until the eggs are cooked to desired consistency.
- Remove from heat and transfer to a plate.
- Serve hot.

Nutritional Information:

- Calories: 220
- Protein: 16g
- Fat: 15g
- Carbohydrates: 4g
- Fiber: 1g
- Sodium: 280mg

- Potassium: 250mg
- Phosphorus: 180mg

MUSHROOM AND SWISS CHEESE BAKED FRITTATA

Time: 35 minutes

Servings: 4

Ingredients:

- 8 egg whites
- 4 whole eggs
- 1 cup sliced mushrooms
- 1/2 cup diced onions
- 1/2 cup diced red bell peppers
- 1/2 cup shredded Swiss cheese
- 2 tablespoons chopped fresh parsley
- 1/4 teaspoon dried thyme
- Cooking spray
- Salt and pepper to taste

Directions:

- Preheat the oven to 350°F (175°C).

- In a bowl, whisk the egg whites and whole eggs until well beaten. Season with salt, pepper, parsley, and dried thyme.
- Heat a non-stick skillet over medium heat and coat with cooking spray.
- Add the mushrooms, onions, and bell peppers to the skillet and sauté until softened.
- Transfer the sautéed vegetables to a greased 9-inch pie dish.
- Pour the beaten eggs over the vegetables in the pie dish.
- Sprinkle the shredded Swiss cheese evenly over the eggs.
- Bake in the preheated oven for 20-25 minutes, or until the eggs are set and the top is lightly golden.
- Remove from the oven and let it cool for a few minutes before slicing.
- Serve warm.

Nutritional Information (per serving):

- Calories: 180
- Protein: 22g
- Fat: 7g
- Carbohydrates: 6g
- Fiber: 1g
- Sodium: 250mg
- Potassium: 280mg
- Phosphorus: 200mg

MEDITERRANEAN EGG MUFFINS

Time: 25 minutes

Servings: 6

Ingredients:

- 6 whole eggs
- 1/2 cup chopped spinach
- 1/4 cup diced tomatoes
- 1/4 cup diced red onions
- 1/4 cup sliced black olives
- 1/4 cup crumbled feta cheese
- 2 tablespoons chopped fresh basil
- Cooking spray
- Salt and pepper to taste

Directions:

- Preheat the oven to 350°F (175°C). Grease a muffin tin with cooking spray.
- In a bowl, whisk the eggs until well beaten. Season with salt and pepper.

- Add the chopped spinach, tomatoes, red onions, black olives, feta cheese, and fresh basil to the bowl. Mix well.
- Divide the mixture evenly among the prepared muffin tin cups.
- Bake in the preheated oven for 15-20 minutes, or until the egg muffins are set and lightly golden on top.
- Remove from the oven and let them cool for a few minutes before removing from the muffin tin.
- Serve warm or refrigerate for later use.

Nutritional Information (per serving, 1 muffin):

- Calories: 90
- Protein: 7g
- Fat: 6g
- Carbohydrates: 2g
- Fiber: 1g
- Sodium: 180mg
- Potassium: 120mg
- Phosphorus: 90mg

BROCCOLI AND CHEDDAR EGG CASSEROLE

Time: 50 minutes

Servings: 6

Ingredients:

- 8 whole eggs
- 1 cup chopped broccoli florets
- 1/2 cup diced onions
- 1/2 cup shredded cheddar cheese
- 1/4 cup chopped fresh parsley
- 1/2 teaspoon garlic powder
- 1/4 teaspoon dried thyme
- Cooking spray
- Salt and pepper to taste

Directions:

- Preheat the oven to 375°F (190°C). Grease a baking dish with cooking spray.
- In a bowl, whisk the eggs until well beaten. Season with salt, pepper, garlic powder, and dried thyme.
- Add the chopped broccoli florets, diced onions, shredded cheddar cheese, and chopped parsley to the bowl. Mix well.
- Pour the mixture into the prepared baking dish.
- Bake in the preheated oven for 30-35 minutes, or until the eggs are set and the top is golden.
- Remove from the oven and let it cool for a few minutes before slicing.

- Serve warm.

Nutritional Information (per serving):

- Calories: 180
- Protein: 13g
- Fat: 12g
- Carbohydrates: 4g
- Fiber: 1g
- Sodium: 220mg
- Potassium: 200mg
- Phosphorus: 150mg

WHOLESOME SMOOTHIES AND FRESH FRUIT IDEAS:

BERRY BLAST SMOOTHIE

Time: 5 minutes

Servings: 2

Ingredients:

- 1 cup unsweetened almond milk

- 1 cup frozen mixed berries (strawberries, blueberries, raspberries)
- 1/2 small avocado
- 1 tablespoon chia seeds
- 1/2 teaspoon vanilla extract
- Ice cubes (optional, for desired thickness)

Directions:

- In a blender, combine almond milk, frozen mixed berries, avocado, chia seeds, and vanilla extract.
- Blend on high speed until smooth and creamy.
- If desired, add ice cubes and blend again for a thicker consistency.
- Pour into glasses and serve immediately.

Nutritional Information (per serving):

- Calories: 120
- Total Fat: 7g
- Sodium: 20mg
- Potassium: 250mg
- Carbohydrates: 14g
- Fiber: 8g
- Sugar: 4g
- Protein: 3g

GREEN POWER SMOOTHIE

Time: 5 minutes

Servings: 2

Ingredients:

- 1 cup unsweetened almond milk
- 1 cup fresh spinach
- 1 small cucumber, peeled and chopped
- 1/2 medium green apple, cored and chopped
- 1/4 ripe avocado
- 1 tablespoon fresh lemon juice
- Ice cubes (optional, for desired thickness)

Directions:

- In a blender, combine almond milk, fresh spinach, cucumber, green apple, avocado, and lemon juice.
- Blend on high speed until smooth and well combined.
- If desired, add ice cubes and blend again for a cooler texture.
- Pour into glasses and serve immediately.

Nutritional Information (per serving):

- Calories: 90
- Total Fat: 5g
- Sodium: 30mg
- Potassium: 430mg
- Carbohydrates: 11g
- Fiber: 5g
- Sugar: 4g
- Protein: 2g

TROPICAL PARADISE SMOOTHIE

Time: 5 minutes

Servings: 2

Ingredients:

- 1 cup unsweetened coconut milk
- 1/2 cup frozen pineapple chunks
- 1/2 cup frozen mango chunks
- 1/4 cup unsweetened shredded coconut
- 1/2 ripe banana
- 1 tablespoon lime juice
- Ice cubes (optional, for desired thickness)

Directions:

- In a blender, combine coconut milk, frozen pineapple chunks, frozen mango chunks, shredded coconut, banana, and lime juice.
- Blend on high speed until smooth and creamy.
- If desired, add ice cubes and blend again for a cooler consistency.
- Pour into glasses and serve immediately.

Nutritional Information (per serving):

- Calories: 150
- Total Fat: 8g
- Sodium: 10mg
- Potassium: 380mg
- Carbohydrates: 21g
- Fiber: 4g
- Sugar: 13g
- Protein: 1g

KIWI AND SPINACH SMOOTHIE

Time: 5 minutes

Servings: 2

Ingredients:

- 1 cup unsweetened almond milk
- 2 kiwis, peeled and chopped
- 1 cup fresh spinach
- 1 tablespoon chia seeds
- 1/2 teaspoon honey (optional)
- Ice cubes (optional, for desired thickness)

Directions:

- In a blender, combine almond milk, kiwis, fresh spinach, chia seeds, and honey (if using).
- Blend on high speed until smooth and well blended.
- If desired, add ice cubes and blend again for a chilled texture.
- Pour into glasses and serve immediately.

Nutritional Information (per serving):

- Calories: 110
- Total Fat: 4g
- Sodium: 30mg
- Potassium: 440mg
- Carbohydrates: 16g
- Fiber: 6g
- Sugar: 7g

- Protein: 3g

WATERMELON LIME REFRESHER

Time: 5 minutes

Servings: 2

Ingredients:

- 2 cups cubed seedless watermelon
- Juice of 1 lime
- 1/2 cup unsweetened coconut water
- Fresh mint leaves for garnish (optional)
- Ice cubes (optional, for desired thickness)

Directions:

- In a blender, combine watermelon cubes, lime juice, and coconut water.
- Blend on high speed until smooth and refreshing.
- If desired, add ice cubes and blend again for a cooler sensation.
- Pour into glasses, garnish with fresh mint leaves (if using), and serve immediately.

Nutritional Information (per serving):

- Calories: 50
- Total Fat: 0g
- Sodium: 10mg
- Potassium: 210mg
- Carbohydrates: 13g
- Fiber: 1g
- Sugar: 10g
- Protein: 1g

CHAPTER 3: NOURISHING SOUPS AND SALADS FOR DIABETIC RENAL HEALTH

VEGETABLE BROTHS AND CLEAR SOUPS:

CLEAR CHICKEN BROTH WITH VEGETABLES

Time: 1 hour

Servings: 4

Ingredients:

- 4 cups low-sodium chicken broth
- 1 small onion, chopped
- 2 carrots, peeled and sliced
- 2 celery stalks, sliced
- 1 small zucchini, sliced
- 1 cup green beans, trimmed and cut into small pieces
- 1 teaspoon dried thyme
- Salt and pepper to taste

Directions:

- In a large pot, bring the chicken broth to a boil over medium heat.
- Add the chopped onion, sliced carrots, sliced celery, zucchini, green beans, dried thyme, salt, and pepper.
- Reduce the heat to low and let the soup simmer for 30-40 minutes until the vegetables are tender.
- Remove from heat and let it cool slightly.
- Using a fine-mesh strainer, strain the broth to remove the vegetables. Discard the vegetables or save them for another use.
- Serve the clear chicken broth hot and season with additional salt and pepper if desired.

Nutritional Information per Serving:

- Calories: 50
- Protein: 6g
- Carbohydrates: 6g
- Fat: 1g
- Sodium: 150mg
- Potassium: 250mg
- Phosphorus: 30mg

GARDEN VEGETABLE SOUP

Time: 45 minutes

Servings: 6

Ingredients:

- 4 cups low-sodium vegetable broth
- 1 small onion, chopped
- 2 cloves garlic, minced
- 2 carrots, peeled and diced
- 2 celery stalks, diced
- 1 zucchini, diced
- 1 cup green beans, trimmed and cut into small pieces
- 1 cup diced tomatoes (fresh or canned)
- 1 teaspoon dried basil
- 1 teaspoon dried oregano
- Salt and pepper to taste

Directions:

- In a large pot, heat the vegetable broth over medium heat.
- Add the chopped onion and minced garlic. Sauté for 2-3 minutes until fragrant.
- Add the diced carrots, diced celery, zucchini, green beans, diced tomatoes, dried basil, dried oregano, salt, and pepper.

- Stir well to combine, then cover the pot and let the soup simmer for 30-40 minutes until the vegetables are tender.
- Adjust the seasoning with salt and pepper if needed.
- Serve the garden vegetable soup hot.

Nutritional Information per Serving:

- Calories: 70
- Protein: 3g
- Carbohydrates: 15g
- Fat: 0.5g
- Sodium: 100mg
- Potassium: 350mg
- Phosphorus: 45mg

TOMATO BASIL SOUP

Time: 1 hour

Servings: 4

Ingredients:

- 2 pounds ripe tomatoes, quartered
- 1 small onion, chopped
- 2 cloves garlic, minced

- 2 cups low-sodium vegetable broth
- 1/4 cup fresh basil leaves, chopped
- 1 tablespoon olive oil
- Salt and pepper to taste

Directions:

- Preheat the oven to 400°F (200°C).
- Place the quartered tomatoes on a baking sheet and drizzle them with olive oil. Roast in the oven for 25-30 minutes until the tomatoes are soft and slightly caramelized.
- In a large pot, heat the olive oil over medium heat. Add the chopped onion and minced garlic, and sauté until translucent.
- Add the roasted tomatoes, vegetable broth, fresh basil leaves, salt, and pepper to the pot. Stir well to combine.
- Bring the mixture to a boil, then reduce the heat and let it simmer for 20-30 minutes.
- Using an immersion blender or a regular blender, puree the soup until smooth.
- Return the soup to the pot and reheat if necessary.
- Serve the tomato basil soup hot, garnished with a few fresh basil leaves.

Nutritional Information per Serving:

- Calories: 90

- Protein: 2g
- Carbohydrates: 15g
- Fat: 3g
- Sodium: 150mg
- Potassium: 500mg
- Phosphorus: 35mg

MUSHROOM CONSOMMÉ

Time: 1 hour

Servings: 4

Ingredients:

- 4 cups low-sodium vegetable broth
- 1 cup sliced mushrooms (such as button or cremini)
- 1 small onion, chopped
- 2 cloves garlic, minced
- 1 tablespoon olive oil
- 1/2 teaspoon dried thyme
- Salt and pepper to taste

Directions:

- In a large pot, heat the olive oil over medium heat. Add the chopped onion and minced garlic, and sauté until translucent.

- Add the sliced mushrooms to the pot and cook for another 5 minutes until they start to release their juices.

- Pour the vegetable broth into the pot and add the dried thyme, salt, and pepper.

- Bring the mixture to a boil, then reduce the heat and let it simmer for 30-40 minutes to allow the flavors to meld together.

- Using a fine-mesh strainer lined with cheesecloth or a coffee filter, strain the consommé to remove any solids.

- Return the consommé to the pot and reheat if necessary.

- Serve the mushroom consommé hot.

Nutritional Information per Serving:

- Calories: 40
- Protein: 2g
- Carbohydrates: 5g
- Fat: 2g
- Sodium: 100mg
- Potassium: 180mg
- Phosphorus: 30mg

CABBAGE AND CARROT CLEAR SOUP

Time: 40 minutes

Servings: 4

Ingredients:

- 4 cups low-sodium vegetable broth
- 2 cups shredded cabbage
- 2 carrots, peeled and thinly sliced
- 1 small onion, chopped
- 2 cloves garlic, minced
- 1 tablespoon olive oil
- 1/2 teaspoon dried thyme
- Salt and pepper to taste

Directions:

- In a large pot, heat the olive oil over medium heat. Add the chopped onion and minced garlic, and sauté until translucent.
- Add the shredded cabbage and sliced carrots to the pot, and cook for 5 minutes until slightly softened.
- Pour the vegetable broth into the pot and add the dried thyme, salt, and pepper.
- Bring the mixture to a boil, then reduce the heat and let it simmer for 25-30 minutes until the vegetables are tender.
- Adjust the seasoning with salt and pepper if needed.

- Serve the cabbage and carrot clear soup hot.

Nutritional Information per Serving:

- Calories: 50
- Protein: 2g
- Carbohydrates: 8g
- Fat: 2g
- Sodium: 120mg
- Potassium: 200mg
- Phosphorus: 35mg

HEARTY BEAN SOUPS WITH REDUCED SODIUM:

TUSCAN WHITE BEAN SOUP

Time: 1 hour

Servings: 4

Ingredients:

- 1 tablespoon olive oil
- 1 onion, diced
- 2 cloves garlic, minced

- 2 carrots, diced

- 2 celery stalks, diced

- 1 can (15 ounces) low-sodium white beans, drained and rinsed

- 4 cups low-sodium vegetable broth

- 1 teaspoon dried rosemary

- 1 teaspoon dried thyme

- Salt and pepper to taste

- Fresh parsley, chopped (for garnish)

Directions:

- In a large pot, heat the olive oil over medium heat. Add the onion and garlic and sauté until the onion becomes translucent.

- Add the carrots and celery to the pot and cook for another 5 minutes, stirring occasionally.

- Add the white beans, vegetable broth, dried rosemary, dried thyme, salt, and pepper. Stir well to combine.

- Bring the soup to a boil, then reduce the heat to low and let it simmer for 30-40 minutes, or until the vegetables are tender.

- Using an immersion blender or a countertop blender, puree a portion of the soup to create a creamy consistency while still leaving some whole beans and vegetables.

- Adjust the seasoning if needed. Serve hot, garnished with fresh parsley.

Nutritional Information (per serving):

- Calories: 180
- Protein: 8g
- Fat: 4g
- Carbohydrates: 30g
- Fiber: 8g
- Sodium: 120mg
- Potassium: 350mg
- Phosphorus: 150mg

LENTIL AND VEGETABLE SOUP

Time: 45 minutes

Servings: 6

Ingredients:

- 1 tablespoon olive oil
- 1 onion, diced
- 2 cloves garlic, minced
- 2 carrots, diced
- 2 celery stalks, diced
- 1 cup dried green lentils, rinsed

- 4 cups low-sodium vegetable broth
- 1 can (14 ounces) diced tomatoes (no salt added)
- 1 teaspoon dried thyme
- 1 teaspoon paprika
- Salt and pepper to taste
- Fresh parsley, chopped (for garnish)

Directions:

- In a large pot, heat the olive oil over medium heat. Add the onion and garlic, and sauté until the onion becomes translucent.
- Add the carrots and celery to the pot and cook for another 5 minutes, stirring occasionally.
- Add the lentils, vegetable broth, diced tomatoes (with their juices), dried thyme, paprika, salt, and pepper. Stir well to combine.
- Bring the soup to a boil, then reduce the heat to low and let it simmer for 30-35 minutes, or until the lentils are tender.
- Adjust the seasoning if needed. Serve hot, garnished with fresh parsley.

Nutritional Information (per serving):

- Calories: 180
- Protein: 10g
- Fat: 3g

- Carbohydrates: 30g
- Fiber: 10g
- Sodium: 120mg
- Potassium: 400mg
- Phosphorus: 200mg

BLACK BEAN AND VEGETABLE CHILI

Time: 1 hour

Servings: 6

Ingredients:

- 1 tablespoon olive oil
- 1 onion, diced
- 2 cloves garlic, minced
- 1 red bell pepper, diced
- 1 green bell pepper, diced
- 1 zucchini, diced
- 1 can (15 ounces) low-sodium black beans, drained and rinsed
- 1 can (14 ounces) diced tomatoes (no salt added)
- 2 cups low-sodium vegetable broth
- 1 tablespoon chili powder
- 1 teaspoon cumin

- Salt and pepper to taste
- Fresh cilantro, chopped (for garnish)

Directions:

- In a large pot, heat the olive oil over medium heat. Add the onion and garlic, and sauté until the onion becomes translucent.
- Add the bell peppers and zucchini to the pot and cook for another 5 minutes, stirring occasionally.
- Add the black beans, diced tomatoes, vegetable broth, chili powder, cumin, salt, and pepper. Stir well to combine.
- Bring the chili to a boil, then reduce the heat to low and let it simmer for 40-45 minutes, allowing the flavors to meld together.
- Adjust the seasoning if needed. Serve hot, garnished with fresh cilantro.

Nutritional Information (per serving):

- Calories: 160
- Protein: 8g
- Fat: 3g
- Carbohydrates: 28g
- Fiber: 10g
- Sodium: 130mg
- Potassium: 400mg
- Phosphorus: 180mg

MINESTRONE SOUP WITH KIDNEY BEANS

Time: 50 minutes

Servings: 6

Ingredients:

- 1 tablespoon olive oil
- 1 onion, diced
- 2 cloves garlic, minced
- 2 carrots, diced
- 2 celery stalks, diced
- 1 can (15 ounces) low-sodium kidney beans, drained and rinsed
- 4 cups low-sodium vegetable broth
- 1 can (14 ounces) diced tomatoes (no salt added)
- 1 teaspoon dried basil
- 1 teaspoon dried oregano
- Salt and pepper to taste
- Whole wheat pasta, cooked (optional)
- Fresh basil, chopped (for garnish)

Directions:

- In a large pot, heat the olive oil over medium heat. Add the onion and garlic, and sauté until the onion becomes translucent.
- Add the carrots and celery to the pot and cook for another 5 minutes, stirring occasionally.
- Add the kidney beans, vegetable broth, diced tomatoes (with their juices), dried basil, dried oregano, salt, and pepper. Stir well to combine.
- Bring the soup to a boil, then reduce the heat to low and let it simmer for 30-35 minutes, allowing the flavors to meld together.
- If desired, add cooked whole wheat pasta to the soup just before serving.
- Adjust the seasoning if needed. Serve hot, garnished with fresh basil.

Nutritional Information (per serving):

- Calories: 160
- Protein: 8g
- Fat: 3g
- Carbohydrates: 28g
- Fiber: 10g
- Sodium: 130mg
- Potassium: 400mg
- Phosphorus: 180mg

SPLIT PEA AND HAM SOUP (USING REDUCED-SODIUM HAM)

Time: 1 hour 30 minutes

Servings: 6

Ingredients:

- 1 tablespoon olive oil
- 1 onion, diced
- 2 cloves garlic, minced
- 2 carrots, diced
- 2 celery stalks, diced
- 1 cup dried split peas, rinsed
- 4 cups low-sodium vegetable broth
- 1 cup reduced-sodium ham, diced
- 1 bay leaf
- Salt and pepper to taste
- Fresh parsley, chopped (for garnish)

Directions:

- In a large pot, heat the olive oil over medium heat. Add the onion and garlic, and sauté until the onion becomes translucent.

- Add the carrots and celery to the pot and cook for another 5 minutes, stirring occasionally.
- Add the split peas, vegetable broth, diced ham, bay leaf, salt, and pepper. Stir well to combine.
- Bring the soup to a boil, then reduce the heat to low and let it simmer for 1 hour to 1 hour 15 minutes, or until the split peas are tender.
- Remove the bay leaf from the soup. Adjust the seasoning if needed. Serve hot, garnished with fresh parsley.

Nutritional Information (per serving):

- Calories: 180
- Protein: 10g
- Fat: 3g
- Carbohydrates: 30g
- Fiber: 10g
- Sodium: 160mg
- Potassium: 400mg
- Phosphorus: 180mg

REFRESHING SALADS WITH KIDNEY-FRIENDLY INGREDIENTS:

MEDITERRANEAN QUINOA SALAD

Time: 30 minutes

Servings: 4

Ingredients:

- 1 cup cooked quinoa
- 1 cup cucumber, diced
- 1 cup cherry tomatoes, halved
- 1/4 cup Kalamata olives, pitted and sliced
- 1/4 cup red onion, finely chopped
- 2 tablespoons fresh parsley, chopped
- 2 tablespoons fresh mint, chopped
- 2 tablespoons lemon juice
- 1 tablespoon extra-virgin olive oil
- Salt and pepper to taste

Directions:

- In a large mixing bowl, combine the cooked quinoa, cucumber, cherry tomatoes, Kalamata olives, red onion, parsley, and mint.
- In a small bowl, whisk together the lemon juice, olive oil, salt, and pepper.
- Pour the dressing over the quinoa mixture and toss until well combined.

- Adjust the seasoning to taste.
- Refrigerate for at least 30 minutes before serving to allow the flavors to meld.
- Serve chilled and enjoy!

Nutritional Information (per serving):

- Calories: 160
- Carbohydrates: 21g
- Protein: 4g
- Fat: 7g
- Sodium: 100mg
- Potassium: 220mg
- Phosphorus: 80mg

ARUGULA AND WATERMELON SALAD

Time: 15 minutes

Servings: 4

Ingredients:

- 4 cups arugula
- 2 cups watermelon, cubed
- 1/4 cup crumbled feta cheese

- 2 tablespoons sliced almonds
- 2 tablespoons balsamic vinegar
- 1 tablespoon extra-virgin olive oil

Directions:

- In a large salad bowl, combine the arugula, watermelon cubes, crumbled feta cheese, and sliced almonds.
- In a small bowl, whisk together the balsamic vinegar and olive oil.
- Drizzle the dressing over the salad and toss gently to coat.
- Serve immediately and enjoy!

Nutritional Information (per serving):

- Calories: 90
- Carbohydrates: 8g
- Protein: 3g
- Fat: 6g
- Sodium: 85mg
- Potassium: 180mg
- Phosphorus: 60mg

CUCUMBER AND TOMATO SALAD WITH LEMON DILL DRESSING

Time: 10 minutes

Servings: 4

Ingredients:

- 2 cucumbers, sliced
- 1 cup cherry tomatoes, halved
- 2 tablespoons fresh dill, chopped
- 2 tablespoons lemon juice
- 1 tablespoon extra-virgin olive oil
- Salt and pepper to taste

Directions:

- In a large bowl, combine the cucumber slices, cherry tomatoes, and fresh dill.
- In a small bowl, whisk together the lemon juice, olive oil, salt, and pepper.
- Pour the dressing over the cucumber and tomato mixture and toss gently to coat.
- Adjust the seasoning to taste.
- Serve immediately and enjoy!

Nutritional Information (per serving):

- Calories: 40

- Carbohydrates: 5g
- Protein: 1g
- Fat: 2g
- Sodium: 5mg
- Potassium: 230mg
- Phosphorus: 20mg

BEET AND ORANGE SALAD WITH GOAT CHEESE

Time: 45 minutes

Servings: 4

Ingredients:

- 2 large beets, roasted, peeled, and diced
- 2 oranges, peeled and segmented
- 2 cups mixed salad greens
- 2 tablespoons crumbled goat cheese
- 2 tablespoons chopped walnuts
- 1 tablespoon balsamic vinegar
- 1 tablespoon extra-virgin olive oil

Directions:

- In a large salad bowl, combine the diced beets, orange segments, mixed salad greens, crumbled goat cheese, and chopped walnuts.
- In a small bowl, whisk together the balsamic vinegar and olive oil.
- Drizzle the dressing over the salad and toss gently to coat.
- Serve immediately and enjoy!

Nutritional Information (per serving):

- Calories: 120
- Carbohydrates: 12g
- Protein: 4g
- Fat: 7g
- Sodium: 85mg
- Potassium: 350mg
- Phosphorus: 80mg

KALE AND BERRY SALAD WITH BALSAMIC VINAIGRETTE

Time: 20 minutes

Servings: 4

Ingredients:

- 4 cups chopped kale leaves
- 1 cup mixed berries (strawberries, blueberries, raspberries)
- 1/4 cup chopped pecans
- 2 tablespoons crumbled feta cheese
- 2 tablespoons balsamic vinegar
- 1 tablespoon extra-virgin olive oil

Directions:

- In a large salad bowl, combine the chopped kale leaves, mixed berries, chopped pecans, and crumbled feta cheese.
- In a small bowl, whisk together the balsamic vinegar and olive oil.
- Drizzle the dressing over the salad and toss gently to coat.
- Allow the salad to sit for a few minutes to allow the kale to soften.
- Serve immediately and enjoy!

Nutritional Information (per serving):

- Calories: 120
- Carbohydrates: 11g
- Protein: 4g
- Fat: 8g

- Sodium: 85mg
- Potassium: 370mg
- Phosphorus: 90mg

CHAPTER 4: DIABETIC RENAL LUNCH AND DINNER IDEAS

LEAN PROTEIN OPTIONS FOR KIDNEY AND DIABETES CARE:

GRILLED CHICKEN BREAST WITH HERBED QUINOA

Time: 40 minutes

Servings: 4

Ingredients:

- 4 boneless, skinless chicken breasts
- 1 tablespoon olive oil
- 1 teaspoon dried basil
- 1 teaspoon dried oregano
- 1 teaspoon dried thyme
- 1 teaspoon garlic powder
- 1/2 teaspoon salt
- 1/4 teaspoon black pepper

For the Herbed Quinoa:

- 1 cup quinoa, rinsed
- 2 cups low-sodium chicken or vegetable broth
- 1 teaspoon dried parsley
- 1/2 teaspoon dried basil
- 1/2 teaspoon dried thyme
- 1/4 teaspoon garlic powder
- 1/4 teaspoon salt
- 1/4 teaspoon black pepper

Directions:

- Preheat the grill to medium-high heat.
- In a small bowl, mix together dried basil, dried oregano, dried thyme, garlic powder, salt, and black pepper to create the seasoning blend.
- Rub the chicken breasts with olive oil and then sprinkle the seasoning blend evenly over both sides of the chicken.
- Place the chicken on the preheated grill and cook for about 6-8 minutes per side or until the internal temperature reaches 165°F (74°C). Remove from the grill and let it rest for a few minutes before serving.
- While the chicken is grilling, prepare the herbed quinoa. In a medium saucepan, bring the chicken or vegetable broth to a boil. Add the rinsed quinoa, dried parsley, dried basil, dried thyme, garlic powder, salt, and black pepper. Stir well, reduce the heat

to low, cover, and simmer for 15-20 minutes or until the quinoa is tender and the liquid is absorbed. Fluff the quinoa with a fork.

- Serve the grilled chicken breasts with a side of herbed quinoa. Enjoy!

Nutritional Information (per serving):

- Calories: 310
- Protein: 36g
- Carbohydrates: 20g
- Fat: 9g
- Sodium: 220mg
- Potassium: 470mg
- Phosphorus: 320mg

BAKED TURKEY CUTLETS WITH STEAMED BROCCOLI

Time: 35 minutes

Servings: 4

Ingredients:

- 4 turkey cutlets
- 2 tablespoons olive oil
- 1 teaspoon dried rosemary

- 1 teaspoon dried thyme
- 1/2 teaspoon garlic powder
- 1/2 teaspoon paprika
- 1/4 teaspoon salt
- 1/4 teaspoon black pepper

For the Steamed Broccoli:

- 4 cups broccoli florets
- 2 teaspoons lemon juice
- 1/4 teaspoon salt

Directions:

- Preheat the oven to 400°F (200°C).
- Place the turkey cutlets on a baking sheet lined with parchment paper.
- Drizzle olive oil over the turkey cutlets, then sprinkle dried rosemary, dried thyme, garlic powder, paprika, salt, and black pepper evenly on both sides of the cutlets.
- Bake in the preheated oven for about 20-25 minutes or until the turkey is cooked through and reaches an internal temperature of 165°F (74°C).
- While the turkey is baking, steam the broccoli florets. Place the broccoli florets in a steamer basket over a pot of boiling water.

Cover and steam for 5-7 minutes or until the broccoli is tender-crisp. Remove from heat and toss with lemon juice and salt.

- Serve the baked turkey cutlets with a side of steamed broccoli. Enjoy!

Nutritional Information (per serving):

- Calories: 230
- Protein: 30g
- Carbohydrates: 6g
- Fat: 9g
- Sodium: 330mg
- Potassium: 500mg
- Phosphorus: 230mg

LEMON HERB SALMON WITH ROASTED ASPARAGUS

Time: 30 minutes

Servings: 4

Ingredients:

- 4 salmon fillets
- 2 tablespoons lemon juice
- 2 teaspoons olive oil

- 1 teaspoon dried dill
- 1/2 teaspoon dried thyme
- 1/4 teaspoon garlic powder
- 1/4 teaspoon salt
- 1/4 teaspoon black pepper

For the Roasted Asparagus:

- 1 bunch asparagus, trimmed
- 1 teaspoon olive oil
- 1/4 teaspoon salt
- 1/4 teaspoon black pepper

Directions:

- Preheat the oven to 400°F (200°C).
- Place the salmon fillets on a baking sheet lined with parchment paper.
- In a small bowl, whisk together lemon juice, olive oil, dried dill, dried thyme, garlic powder, salt, and black pepper. Drizzle the mixture evenly over the salmon fillets.
- Bake in the preheated oven for about 15-20 minutes or until the salmon is cooked through and flakes easily with a fork.
- While the salmon is baking, prepare the roasted asparagus. Place the trimmed asparagus on a separate baking sheet. Drizzle with

olive oil, then sprinkle with salt and black pepper. Toss to coat evenly.

- After 10 minutes of baking the salmon, place the asparagus in the oven and roast for an additional 10-12 minutes or until the asparagus is tender-crisp.
- Serve the lemon herb salmon with roasted asparagus. Enjoy!

Nutritional Information (per serving):

- Calories: 300
- Protein: 34g
- Carbohydrates: 5g
- Fat: 16g
- Sodium: 260mg
- Potassium: 700mg
- Phosphorus: 400mg

TOFU STIR-FRY WITH MIXED VEGETABLES

Time: 25 minutes

Servings: 4

Ingredients:

- 1 tablespoon olive oil

- 1 tablespoon low-sodium soy sauce
- 2 teaspoons cornstarch
- 1/2 teaspoon ground ginger
- 1/4 teaspoon garlic powder
- 1/4 teaspoon black pepper
- 14 ounces firm tofu, drained and cubed
- 1 cup broccoli florets
- 1 cup sliced bell peppers
- 1 cup sliced zucchini
- 1 cup sliced mushrooms
- 1/2 cup sliced carrots
- 2 green onions, sliced

Directions:

- In a small bowl, whisk together olive oil, soy sauce, cornstarch, ground ginger, garlic powder, and black pepper to create the stir-fry sauce.
- Heat a non-stick skillet or wok over medium-high heat. Add the tofu cubes and cook until lightly browned on all sides, about 5-7 minutes. Remove the tofu from the skillet and set aside.
- In the same skillet, add broccoli, bell peppers, zucchini, mushrooms, and carrots. Stir-fry for about 5 minutes or until the vegetables are crisp-tender.

- Return the tofu to the skillet and pour the stir-fry sauce over the tofu and vegetables. Cook for an additional 2-3 minutes, stirring gently to coat everything evenly.
- Sprinkle sliced green onions on top of the stir-fry.
- Serve the tofu stir-fry with mixed vegetables over cooked quinoa or brown rice. Enjoy!

Nutritional Information (per serving):

- Calories: 220
- Protein: 16g
- Carbohydrates: 16g
- Fat: 10g
- Sodium: 250mg
- Potassium: 530mg
- Phosphorus: 190mg

PORK TENDERLOIN WITH SWEET POTATO MASH

Time: 1 hour

Servings: 4

Ingredients:

- 1 pound pork tenderloin

- 2 teaspoons olive oil

- 1 teaspoon dried rosemary

- 1 teaspoon dried thyme

- 1/2 teaspoon garlic powder

- 1/4 teaspoon salt

- 1/4 teaspoon black pepper

For the Sweet Potato Mash:

- 2 large sweet potatoes, peeled and cubed

- 1/4 cup low-sodium chicken or vegetable broth

- 1/2 teaspoon ground cinnamon

- 1/4 teaspoon nutmeg

- 1/4 teaspoon salt

Directions:

- Preheat the oven to 400°F (200°C).

- Rub the pork tenderloin with olive oil, then sprinkle dried rosemary, dried thyme, garlic powder, salt, and black pepper evenly over the pork.

- Place the seasoned pork tenderloin on a baking sheet lined with parchment paper.

- Roast in the preheated oven for about 30-35 minutes or until the internal temperature reaches 145°F (63°C). Remove from the oven and let it rest for a few minutes before slicing.

- While the pork is roasting, prepare the sweet potato mash. Place the cubed sweet potatoes in a large saucepan and cover with water. Bring to a boil, then reduce the heat to medium and simmer for about 15-20 minutes or until the sweet potatoes are tender.

- Drain the sweet potatoes and return them to the saucepan. Add the chicken or vegetable broth, ground cinnamon, nutmeg, and salt. Mash the sweet potatoes until smooth and creamy.

- Slice the roasted pork tenderloin and serve it with a side of sweet potato mash. Enjoy!

Nutritional Information (per serving):

- Calories: 290
- Protein: 27g
- Carbohydrates: 22g
- Fat: 9g
- Sodium: 310mg
- Potassium: 660mg
- Phosphorus: 330mg

FLAVORFUL GRILLED AND BAKED FISH RECIPES:

GRILLED LEMON PEPPER COD

Time: 25 minutes

Servings: 4

Ingredients:

- 4 cod fillets (4-6 ounces each)
- 1 tablespoon lemon zest
- 1 teaspoon black pepper
- 1 teaspoon dried thyme
- 1 teaspoon garlic powder
- 1 tablespoon olive oil
- Lemon wedges for serving

Directions:

- Preheat the grill to medium-high heat.
- In a small bowl, combine the lemon zest, black pepper, dried thyme, and garlic powder.
- Brush the cod fillets with olive oil on both sides.
- Sprinkle the lemon pepper seasoning mixture evenly over the cod fillets.
- Place the cod fillets on the preheated grill and cook for about 4-5 minutes per side, or until the fish flakes easily with a fork and reaches an internal temperature of 145°F (63°C).

- Remove the grilled cod fillets from the heat and let them rest for a few minutes.
- Serve the grilled lemon pepper cod with lemon wedges on the side.

Nutritional Information (per serving):

- Calories: 180
- Protein: 25g
- Fat: 7g
- Carbohydrates: 0g
- Fiber: 0g
- Sodium: 70mg
- Potassium: 490mg
- Phosphorus: 225mg

BAKED GARLIC BUTTER SALMON

Time: 30 minutes

Servings: 4

Ingredients:

- 4 salmon fillets (4-6 ounces each)
- 2 cloves garlic, minced

- 2 tablespoons unsalted butter, melted
- 1 tablespoon chopped fresh dill
- Salt and black pepper to taste
- Lemon wedges for serving

Directions:

- Preheat the oven to 400°F (200°C). Line a baking sheet with parchment paper or foil.
- Place the salmon fillets on the prepared baking sheet.
- In a small bowl, mix together the minced garlic, melted butter, chopped fresh dill, salt, and black pepper.
- Brush the garlic butter mixture evenly over the salmon fillets.
- Bake the salmon in the preheated oven for about 15-20 minutes, or until the fish flakes easily with a fork and reaches an internal temperature of 145°F (63°C).
- Remove the baked garlic butter salmon from the oven and let it rest for a few minutes.
- Serve the salmon with lemon wedges on the side.

Nutritional Information (per serving):

- Calories: 280
- Protein: 25g
- Fat: 19g
- Carbohydrates: 1g

- Fiber: 0g
- Sodium: 70mg
- Potassium: 520mg
- Phosphorus: 275mg

CITRUS HERB TILAPIA

Time: 25 minutes

Servings: 4

Ingredients:

- 4 tilapia fillets (4-6 ounces each)
- 1 tablespoon lemon juice
- 1 tablespoon lime juice
- 1 tablespoon orange juice
- 1 teaspoon dried thyme
- 1 teaspoon dried oregano
- 1 teaspoon paprika
- Salt and black pepper to taste
- 1 tablespoon olive oil
- Lemon wedges for serving

Directions:

- Preheat the oven to 375°F (190°C). Line a baking dish with parchment paper or foil.
- Place the tilapia fillets in the prepared baking dish.
- In a small bowl, whisk together the lemon juice, lime juice, orange juice, dried thyme, dried oregano, paprika, salt, black pepper, and olive oil.
- Pour the citrus herb marinade over the tilapia fillets, ensuring they are evenly coated.
- Bake the tilapia in the preheated oven for about 15-20 minutes, or until the fish flakes easily with a fork and reaches an internal temperature of 145°F (63°C).
- Remove the citrus herb tilapia from the oven and let it rest for a few minutes.
- Serve the tilapia with lemon wedges on the side.

Nutritional Information (per serving):

- Calories: 150
- Protein: 26g
- Fat: 4g
- Carbohydrates: 2g
- Fiber: 0g
- Sodium: 75mg
- Potassium: 460mg
- Phosphorus: 275mg

TERIYAKI GLAZED MAHI-MAHI

Time: 30 minutes

Servings: 4

Ingredients:

- 4 mahi-mahi fillets (4-6 ounces each)
- 2 tablespoons reduced-sodium soy sauce
- 2 tablespoons water
- 2 tablespoons unsweetened pineapple juice
- 1 tablespoon low-sodium teriyaki sauce
- 1 tablespoon honey
- 1 teaspoon minced ginger
- 1 teaspoon minced garlic
- 1 teaspoon cornstarch (optional, for thickening the glaze)
- Sesame seeds for garnish (optional)
- Chopped green onions for garnish (optional)

Directions:

- Preheat the oven to 400°F (200°C). Line a baking sheet with parchment paper or foil.
- Place the mahi-mahi fillets on the prepared baking sheet.

- In a small saucepan, whisk together the reduced-sodium soy sauce, water, pineapple juice, teriyaki sauce, honey, minced ginger, and minced garlic.
- Bring the sauce to a simmer over medium heat. If desired, mix the cornstarch with a little water to create a slurry, then add it to the sauce to thicken it. Stir well.
- Brush the teriyaki glaze over the mahi-mahi fillets, reserving some glaze for serving.
- Bake the mahi-mahi in the preheated oven for about 15-20 minutes, or until the fish flakes easily with a fork and reaches an internal temperature of 145°F (63°C).
- Remove the teriyaki glazed mahi-mahi from the oven and let it rest for a few minutes.
- Serve the mahi-mahi with the reserved teriyaki glaze drizzled on top. Garnish with sesame seeds and chopped green onions, if desired.

Nutritional Information (per serving):

- Calories: 190
- Protein: 33g
- Fat: 2g
- Carbohydrates: 8g
- Fiber: 0g
- Sodium: 320mg

- Potassium: 580mg
- Phosphorus: 310mg

HERB-CRUSTED HALIBUT

Time: 25 minutes

Servings: 4

Ingredients:

- 4 halibut fillets (4-6 ounces each)
- 2 tablespoons chopped fresh parsley
- 2 tablespoons chopped fresh dill
- 1 tablespoon grated lemon zest
- 1 teaspoon minced garlic
- 1 teaspoon olive oil
- Salt and black pepper to taste
- Lemon wedges for serving

Directions:

- Preheat the oven to 400°F (200°C). Line a baking sheet with parchment paper or foil.
- Place the halibut fillets on the prepared baking sheet.

- In a small bowl, combine the chopped fresh parsley, chopped fresh dill, grated lemon zest, minced garlic, olive oil, salt, and black pepper.
- Press the herb mixture onto the top of each halibut fillet, forming a crust.
- Bake the halibut in the preheated oven for about 12-15 minutes, or until the fish flakes easily with a fork and reaches an internal temperature of 145°F (63°C).
- Remove the herb-crusted halibut from the oven and let it rest for a few minutes.
- Serve the halibut with lemon wedges on the side.

Nutritional Information (per serving):

- Calories: 160
- Protein: 34g
- Fat: 2g
- Carbohydrates: 0g
- Fiber: 0g
- Sodium: 95mg
- Potassium: 800mg
- Phosphorus: 350mg

TASTY VEGETABLE STIR-FRIES AND STEWS:

GINGER GARLIC VEGETABLE STIR-FRY

Time. 25 minutes

Servings: 4

Ingredients:

- 1 tablespoon olive oil
- 2 cloves garlic, minced
- 1 tablespoon fresh ginger, grated
- 1 medium onion, thinly sliced
- 2 cups broccoli florets
- 1 red bell pepper, thinly sliced
- 1 small zucchini, sliced
- 1 cup snap peas
- 2 tablespoons low-sodium soy sauce
- 1 tablespoon rice vinegar
- 1 teaspoon sesame oil
- 1/4 teaspoon black pepper
- 2 green onions, sliced (for garnish)

Directions:

- Heat the olive oil in a large skillet or wok over medium heat.

- Add the minced garlic and grated ginger to the skillet. Cook for 1-2 minutes until fragrant.
- Add the sliced onion and cook for another 2-3 minutes until the onion is translucent.
- Add the broccoli florets, red bell pepper, zucchini, and snap peas to the skillet. Stir-fry for 4-5 minutes until the vegetables are tender-crisp.
- In a small bowl, whisk together the low-sodium soy sauce, rice vinegar, sesame oil, and black pepper.
- Pour the sauce over the vegetables in the skillet and toss to coat evenly. Cook for an additional 1-2 minutes to heat through.
- Remove from heat and garnish with sliced green onions.
- Serve the Ginger Garlic Vegetable Stir-Fry over cooked brown rice or quinoa, if desired.

Nutritional Information per serving:

- Calories: 105kcal
- Carbohydrates: 11g
- Protein: 4g
- Fat: 6g
- Sodium: 143mg
- Potassium: 298mg
- Phosphorus: 73mg

SPICY TOFU AND VEGETABLE STIR-FRY

Time: 30 minutes

Servings: 4

Ingredients:

- 1 tablespoon olive oil
- 1 block (14oz) firm tofu, drained and cut into cubes
- 2 cloves garlic, minced
- 1 tablespoon fresh ginger, grated
- 1 small onion, thinly sliced
- 1 red bell pepper, thinly sliced
- 1 medium carrot, julienned
- 1 cup snow peas
- 2 tablespoons low-sodium soy sauce
- 1 tablespoon rice vinegar
- 1 tablespoon sriracha sauce (adjust to taste)
- 1 teaspoon sesame oil
- 1/4 teaspoon black pepper
- 2 green onions, sliced (for garnish)

Directions:

- Heat the olive oil in a large skillet or wok over medium heat.
- Add the tofu cubes to the skillet and cook for 5-6 minutes, stirring occasionally, until lightly browned. Remove tofu from the skillet and set aside.
- In the same skillet, add the minced garlic and grated ginger. Cook for 1-2 minutes until fragrant.
- Add the sliced onion, red bell pepper, carrot, and snow peas to the skillet. Stir-fry for 4-5 minutes until the vegetables are crisp-tender.
- In a small bowl, whisk together the low-sodium soy sauce, rice vinegar, sriracha sauce, sesame oil, and black pepper.
- Return the tofu to the skillet and pour the sauce over the tofu and vegetables. Toss to coat evenly and cook for an additional 1-2 minutes to heat through.
- Remove from heat and garnish with sliced green onions.
- Serve the Spicy Tofu and Vegetable Stir-Fry over cooked quinoa or brown rice, if desired.

Nutritional Information per serving:

- Calories: 163kcal
- Carbohydrates: 12g
- Protein: 9g
- Fat: 9g
- Sodium: 190mg

- Potassium: 288mg
- Phosphorus: 119mg

RATATOUILLE STEW WITH CHICKPEAS

Time: 45 minutes

Servings: 6

Ingredients:

- 2 tablespoons olive oil
- 1 medium onion, chopped
- 3 cloves garlic, minced
- 1 medium eggplant, cubed
- 1 medium zucchini, sliced
- 1 red bell pepper, chopped
- 1 yellow bell pepper, chopped
- 1 can (14oz) diced tomatoes, no added salt
- 1 can (14oz) chickpeas, drained and rinsed
- 1 tablespoon tomato paste
- 1 teaspoon dried basil
- 1 teaspoon dried oregano
- 1/2 teaspoon dried thyme
- 1/4 teaspoon black pepper

- Fresh basil leaves (for garnish)

Directions:

- Heat the olive oil in a large pot or Dutch oven over medium heat.
- Add the chopped onion and minced garlic to the pot. Cook for 3-4 minutes until the onion is translucent and the garlic is fragrant.
- Add the cubed eggplant, sliced zucchini, and chopped bell peppers to the pot. Stir well to combine.
- Cook the vegetables for 5-6 minutes until they start to soften.
- Add the diced tomatoes, chickpeas, tomato paste, dried basil, dried oregano, dried thyme, and black pepper to the pot. Stir to combine all the ingredients.
- Reduce the heat to low, cover the pot, and simmer for 25-30 minutes, stirring occasionally, until the vegetables are tender and the flavors are well combined.
- Remove from heat and garnish with fresh basil leaves.
- Serve the Ratatouille Stew with Chickpeas as a main dish or alongside cooked whole grain pasta or crusty bread.

Nutritional Information per serving:

- Calories: 172kcal
- Carbohydrates: 28g
- Protein: 7g

- Fat: 5g
- Sodium: 16mg
- Potassium: 488mg
- Phosphorus: 128mg

COCONUT CURRY VEGETABLE STEW

Time: 40 minutes

Servings: 4

Ingredients:

- 1 tablespoon olive oil
- 1 medium onion, chopped
- 2 cloves garlic, minced
- 1 tablespoon fresh ginger, grated
- 1 tablespoon curry powder
- 1 teaspoon ground cumin
- 1 teaspoon ground coriander
- 1/2 teaspoon turmeric
- 1/4 teaspoon cayenne pepper (optional)
- 1 medium sweet potato, peeled and cubed
- 1 medium carrot, sliced
- 1 red bell pepper, chopped

- 1 can (14oz) light coconut milk
- 1 cup low-sodium vegetable broth
- 2 cups broccoli florets
- 1 cup cauliflower florets
- 1 cup green beans, trimmed
- 2 tablespoons fresh cilantro, chopped (for garnish)
- Lime wedges (for serving)

Directions:

- Heat the olive oil in a large pot or Dutch oven over medium heat.
- Add the chopped onion, minced garlic, and grated ginger to the pot. Cook for 3-4 minutes until the onion is translucent and the spices are fragrant.
- Add the curry powder, cumin, coriander, turmeric, and cayenne pepper (if using) to the pot. Stir well to coat the onions and garlic with the spices.
- Add the cubed sweet potato, sliced carrot, and chopped red bell pepper to the pot. Stir to combine.
- Pour in the light coconut milk and low-sodium vegetable broth. Bring the mixture to a boil.
- Reduce the heat to low, cover the pot, and simmer for 15-20 minutes until the sweet potato and carrot are tender.
- Add the broccoli florets, cauliflower florets, and green beans to the pot. Stir well to combine.

- Cover the pot again and simmer for an additional 8-10 minutes until the vegetables are cooked but still crisp.
- Remove from heat and garnish with fresh cilantro.
- Serve the Coconut Curry Vegetable Stew hot with lime wedges for squeezing over the stew.

Nutritional Information per serving:

- Calories: 215kcal
- Carbohydrates: 30g
- Protein: 6g
- Fat: 9g
- Sodium: 98mg
- Potassium: 762mg
- Phosphorus: 133mg

SZECHUAN EGGPLANT STIR-FRY

Time: 30 minutes

Servings: 4

Ingredients:

- 2 tablespoons olive oil
- 2 cloves garlic, minced

- 1 tablespoon fresh ginger, grated
- 2 medium eggplants, cubed
- 1 red bell pepper, thinly sliced
- 1 medium onion, thinly sliced
- 1 tablespoon low-sodium soy sauce
- 1 tablespoon rice vinegar
- 1 tablespoon hoisin sauce (low-sodium)
- 1 teaspoon sesame oil
- 1/2 teaspoon Szechuan peppercorns, crushed
- 1/4 teaspoon red pepper flakes (adjust to taste)
- 2 green onions, sliced (for garnish)

Directions:

- Heat the olive oil in a large skillet or wok over medium heat.
- Add the minced garlic and grated ginger to the skillet. Cook for 1-2 minutes until fragrant.
- Add the cubed eggplants, sliced red bell pepper, and sliced onion to the skillet. Stir-fry for 6-8 minutes until the vegetables are tender.
- In a small bowl, whisk together the low-sodium soy sauce, rice vinegar, hoisin sauce, sesame oil, crushed Szechuan peppercorns, and red pepper flakes.
- Pour the sauce over the vegetables in the skillet and toss to coat evenly. Cook for an additional 1-2 minutes to heat through.

- Remove from heat and garnish with sliced green onions.
- Serve the Szechuan Eggplant Stir-Fry over cooked brown rice or quinoa, if desired.

Nutritional Information per serving:

- Calories: 133kcal
- Carbohydrates: 19g
- Protein: 3g
- Fat: 7g
- Sodium: 153mg
- Potassium: 420mg
- Phosphorus: 57mg

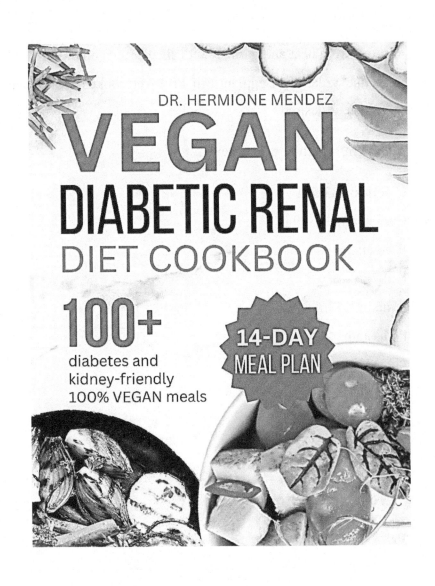

GET ON AMAZON NOW!

CHAPTER 5: KIDNEY-FRIENDLY SIDE DISHES AND SNACKS

LOW-POTASSIUM VEGETABLE MEDLEYS:

ROASTED CAULIFLOWER AND BRUSSELS SPROUTS

Time: 40 minutes

Servings: 4

Ingredients:

- 1 head of cauliflower, cut into florets
- 1 pound Brussels sprouts, trimmed and halved
- 2 tablespoons olive oil
- 1 teaspoon garlic powder
- 1 teaspoon dried thyme
- Salt and pepper, to taste

Directions:

- Preheat the oven to 400°F (200°C) and line a baking sheet with parchment paper.

- In a large bowl, combine the cauliflower florets and Brussels sprouts.
- Drizzle the olive oil over the vegetables and toss to coat them evenly.
- Sprinkle the garlic powder, dried thyme, salt, and pepper over the vegetables and toss again.
- Spread the vegetables in a single layer on the prepared baking sheet.
- Roast in the preheated oven for about 30 minutes or until the vegetables are golden brown and tender, stirring once halfway through.
- Remove from the oven and serve hot.

Nutritional Information (per serving):

- Calories: 110
- Carbohydrates: 11g
- Protein: 5g
- Fat: 7g
- Sodium: 35mg
- Potassium: 520mg
- Phosphorus: 90mg

SAUTÉED ZUCCHINI AND YELLOW SQUASH

Time: 15 minutes

Servings: 4

Ingredients:

- 2 medium zucchini, sliced
- 2 medium yellow squash, sliced
- 1 tablespoon olive oil
- 2 cloves garlic, minced
- 1 teaspoon dried oregano
- Salt and pepper, to taste

Directions:

- Heat the olive oil in a large skillet over medium heat.
- Add the minced garlic and sauté for 1-2 minutes until fragrant.
- Add the sliced zucchini and yellow squash to the skillet.
- Sprinkle with dried oregano, salt, and pepper.
- Cook, stirring occasionally, for about 8-10 minutes or until the vegetables are tender yet still slightly crisp.
- Remove from heat and serve warm.

Nutritional Information (per serving):

- Calories: 50
- Carbohydrates: 6g

- Protein: 2g
- Fat: 3g
- Sodium: 5mg
- Potassium: 400mg
- Phosphorus: 40mg

STEAMED GREEN BEANS WITH LEMON AND ALMONDS

Time: 15 minutes

Servings: 4

Ingredients:

- 1 pound green beans, ends trimmed
- 2 tablespoons slivered almonds
- 1 tablespoon olive oil
- 1 tablespoon fresh lemon juice
- Zest of 1 lemon
- Salt and pepper, to taste

Directions:

- Fill a large pot with about 1 inch of water and bring it to a boil.
- Place the green beans in a steamer basket and set it over the boiling water.

- Cover the pot and steam the green beans for 5-7 minutes or until they are tender yet still vibrant green.
- While the green beans are steaming, heat a small skillet over medium heat.
- Add the slivered almonds to the skillet and toast them, stirring frequently, until golden brown and fragrant.
- In a serving bowl, combine the steamed green beans, toasted almonds, olive oil, lemon juice, lemon zest, salt, and pepper.
- Toss gently to coat the green beans with the dressing.
- Serve immediately.

Nutritional Information (per serving):

- Calories: 70
- Carbohydrates: 8g
- Protein: 3g
- Fat: 4g
- Sodium: 10mg
- Potassium: 250mg
- Phosphorus: 45mg

ROASTED ROOT VEGETABLES (CARROTS, PARSNIPS, AND TURNIPS)

Time: 45 minutes

Servings: 4

Ingredients:

- 2 large carrots, peeled and cut into thick slices
- 2 large parsnips, peeled and cut into thick slices
- 2 small turnips, peeled and cut into wedges
- 2 tablespoons olive oil
- 1 teaspoon dried rosemary
- 1 teaspoon dried thyme
- Salt and pepper, to taste

Directions:

- Preheat the oven to 400°F (200°C) and line a baking sheet with parchment paper.
- In a large bowl, combine the carrot slices, parsnip slices, and turnip wedges.
- Drizzle the olive oil over the vegetables and toss to coat them evenly.
- Sprinkle the dried rosemary, dried thyme, salt, and pepper over the vegetables and toss again.
- Spread the vegetables in a single layer on the prepared baking sheet.

- Roast in the preheated oven for about 35-40 minutes or until the vegetables are golden brown and tender, stirring once halfway through.
- Remove from the oven and serve hot.

Nutritional Information (per serving):

- Calories: 110
- Carbohydrates: 16g
- Protein: 2g
- Fat: 5g
- Sodium: 45mg
- Potassium: 430mg
- Phosphorus: 65mg

GRILLED ASPARAGUS WITH BALSAMIC GLAZE

Time: 15 minutes

Servings: 4

Ingredients:

- 1 pound asparagus spears, ends trimmed
- 1 tablespoon olive oil
- Salt and pepper, to taste

- 2 tablespoons balsamic vinegar

Directions:

- Preheat a grill or grill pan over medium-high heat.
- In a shallow dish, toss the asparagus spears with olive oil, salt, and pepper.
- Place the asparagus on the preheated grill and cook for about 5-7 minutes, turning occasionally, until tender and lightly charred.
- While the asparagus is grilling, heat the balsamic vinegar in a small saucepan over medium heat. Simmer for a few minutes until the vinegar reduces and thickens slightly.
- Transfer the grilled asparagus to a serving platter and drizzle with the balsamic glaze.
- Serve immediately.

Nutritional Information (per serving):

- Calories: 40
- Carbohydrates: 5g
- Protein: 2g
- Fat: 2g
- Sodium: 0mg
- Potassium: 250mg
- Phosphorus: 40mg

CREATIVE WHOLE GRAIN RECIPES FOR SIDES:

QUINOA PILAF WITH MIXED VEGETABLES

Time: 30 minutes

Servings: 4

Ingredients:

- 1 cup quinoa
- 2 cups low-sodium vegetable broth
- 1 tablespoon olive oil
- 1 small onion, diced
- 2 cloves garlic, minced
- 1 cup mixed vegetables (such as bell peppers, carrots, zucchini), diced
- 1/4 teaspoon dried thyme
- Salt and pepper to taste
- Fresh parsley for garnish

Directions:

- Rinse the quinoa thoroughly under cold water.

- In a medium-sized saucepan, bring the vegetable broth to a boil. Add the quinoa, reduce heat to low, cover, and simmer for 15-20 minutes or until the quinoa is tender and the liquid is absorbed.
- In a separate skillet, heat olive oil over medium heat. Add the diced onion and minced garlic, and sauté until the onion becomes translucent.
- Add the mixed vegetables to the skillet and cook for about 5-7 minutes until they are slightly tender.
- Stir in the cooked quinoa and dried thyme. Season with salt and pepper to taste. Cook for an additional 2-3 minutes to allow the flavors to combine.
- Remove from heat and garnish with fresh parsley.
- Serve hot as a main dish or a side dish.

Nutritional Information (per serving):

- Calories: 210
- Carbohydrates: 36g
- Protein: 6g
- Fat: 5g
- Sodium: 60mg
- Potassium: 230mg
- Phosphorus: 115mg

BROWN RICE AND BLACK BEAN SALAD

Time: 25 minutes

Servings: 4

Ingredients:

- 1 cup cooked brown rice
- 1 cup canned low-sodium black beans, rinsed and drained
- 1 small red bell pepper, diced
- 1/2 cup cucumber, diced
- 1/4 cup red onion, finely chopped
- 2 tablespoons fresh cilantro, chopped
- 2 tablespoons fresh lime juice
- 1 tablespoon olive oil
- 1/2 teaspoon ground cumin
- Salt and pepper to taste

Directions:

- In a large mixing bowl, combine the cooked brown rice, black beans, red bell pepper, cucumber, red onion, and cilantro.
- In a separate small bowl, whisk together the lime juice, olive oil, ground cumin, salt, and pepper.

- Pour the dressing over the rice and bean mixture and toss gently to combine.
- Adjust the seasoning if needed.
- Cover and refrigerate for at least 30 minutes to allow the flavors to meld.
- Serve chilled as a refreshing salad.

Nutritional Information (per serving):

- Calories: 190
- Carbohydrates: 33g
- Protein: 6g
- Fat: 4g
- Sodium: 20mg
- Potassium: 275mg
- Phosphorus: 105mg

BARLEY AND MUSHROOM RISOTTO

Time: 45 minutes

Servings: 4

Ingredients:

- 1 cup pearl barley

- 4 cups low-sodium vegetable broth
- 1 tablespoon olive oil
- 1 small onion, diced
- 2 cloves garlic, minced
- 8 ounces mushrooms, sliced
- 1/4 cup grated Parmesan cheese (optional)
- Fresh parsley for garnish
- Salt and pepper to taste

Directions:

- In a medium-sized saucepan, bring the vegetable broth to a boil. Add the pearl barley, reduce heat to low, cover, and simmer for 30-35 minutes or until the barley is tender and the liquid is absorbed.
- In a separate skillet, heat olive oil over medium heat. Add the diced onion and minced garlic, and sauté until the onion becomes translucent.
- Add the sliced mushrooms to the skillet and cook for about 7-10 minutes until they release their juices and are slightly browned.
- Stir in the cooked barley and grated Parmesan cheese (if using). Season with salt and pepper to taste. Cook for an additional 2-3 minutes to allow the flavors to combine.
- Remove from heat and garnish with fresh parsley.
- Serve hot as a satisfying risotto alternative.

Nutritional Information (per serving):

- Calories: 230
- Carbohydrates: 44g
- Protein: 8g
- Fat: 4g
- Sodium: 70mg
- Potassium: 275mg
- Phosphorus: 165mg

WILD RICE WITH CRANBERRIES AND PECANS

Time: 40 minutes

Servings: 4

Ingredients:

- 1 cup wild rice
- 2 cups low-sodium vegetable broth
- 1/4 cup dried cranberries
- 1/4 cup chopped pecans
- 2 tablespoons chopped fresh parsley
- 1 tablespoon olive oil
- 1 tablespoon balsamic vinegar

- Salt and pepper to taste

Directions:

- Rinse the wild rice thoroughly under cold water.
- In a medium-sized saucepan, bring the vegetable broth to a boil. Add the wild rice, reduce heat to low, cover, and simmer for 35-40 minutes or until the rice is tender and the liquid is absorbed.
- In a separate small bowl, whisk together the olive oil, balsamic vinegar, salt, and pepper.
- In a serving bowl, combine the cooked wild rice, dried cranberries, chopped pecans, and fresh parsley.
- Pour the dressing over the rice mixture and toss gently to combine.
- Adjust the seasoning if needed.
- Serve warm as a delightful side dish.

Nutritional Information (per serving):

- Calories: 240
- Carbohydrates: 41g
- Protein: 5g
- Fat: 7g
- Sodium: 30mg
- Potassium: 180mg
- Phosphorus: 125mg

BULGUR WHEAT AND ROASTED VEGETABLE SALAD

Time: 35 minutes

Servings: 4

Ingredients:

- 1 cup bulgur wheat
- 2 cups low-sodium vegetable broth
- 1 small eggplant, diced
- 1 red bell pepper, diced
- 1 zucchini, diced
- 1 tablespoon olive oil
- 2 tablespoons lemon juice
- 1 tablespoon fresh mint, chopped
- Salt and pepper to taste

Directions:

- Preheat the oven to 400°F (200°C).
- In a medium-sized saucepan, bring the vegetable broth to a boil. Add the bulgur wheat, reduce heat to low, cover, and simmer for 15-20 minutes or until the wheat is tender and the liquid is absorbed.

- In a baking dish, toss the diced eggplant, red bell pepper, and zucchini with olive oil, salt, and pepper.
- Roast the vegetables in the preheated oven for 20-25 minutes or until they are tender and slightly browned.
- In a serving bowl, combine the cooked bulgur wheat, roasted vegetables, lemon juice, and fresh mint. Toss gently to combine.
- Adjust the seasoning if needed.
- Serve at room temperature as a satisfying salad.

Nutritional Information (per serving):

- Calories: 210
- Carbohydrates: 39g
- Protein: 5g
- Fat: 5g
- Sodium: 30mg
- Potassium: 325mg
- Phosphorus: 120mg

DIABETIC RENAL SNACKS FOR SUSTAINED ENERGY:

ALMOND BUTTER AND APPLE SLICES

Time: 5 minutes

Servings: 1

Ingredients:

- 1 medium-sized apple
- 1 tablespoon almond butter (unsweetened and low-sodium)

Directions:

- Wash the apple and cut it into thin slices.
- Spread the almond butter evenly on the apple slices.
- Arrange the apple slices on a plate and serve.

Nutritional Information:

- Calories: 150
- Total Fat: 7g
- Sodium: 0mg
- Potassium: 180mg
- Carbohydrates: 20g
- Fiber: 4g
- Sugars: 13g
- Protein: 3g

GREEK YOGURT PARFAIT WITH BERRIES

Time: 10 minutes

Servings: 1

Ingredients:

- 1/2 cup plain Greek yogurt (low-sugar and low-sodium)
- 1/4 cup mixed berries (such as strawberries, blueberries, and raspberries)
- 1 tablespoon chopped nuts (such as almonds or walnuts)

Directions:

- In a serving glass or bowl, layer half of the Greek yogurt.
- Add half of the mixed berries on top of the yogurt layer.
- Repeat the layers with the remaining Greek yogurt and mixed berries.
- Sprinkle the chopped nuts over the top layer.
- Serve immediately or refrigerate until ready to enjoy.

Nutritional Information:

- Calories: 200
- Total Fat: 10g
- Sodium: 40mg
- Potassium: 200mg

- Carbohydrates: 15g
- Fiber: 4g
- Sugars: 8g
- Protein: 15g

CELERY STICKS WITH HUMMUS

Time: 5 minutes

Servings: 1

Ingredients:

- 2 stalks of celery
- 2 tablespoons low-sodium hummus

Directions:

- Wash the celery stalks and cut them into manageable sticks.
- Serve the celery sticks with the hummus for dipping.

Nutritional Information:

- Calories: 70
- Total Fat: 3g
- Sodium: 70mg
- Potassium: 260mg

- Carbohydrates: 8g
- Fiber: 3g
- Sugars: 2g
- Protein: 3g

TRAIL MIX WITH NUTS AND SEEDS

Time: 5 minutes

Servings: 1

Ingredients:

- 1/4 cup mixed nuts (such as almonds, cashews, and peanuts)
- 1 tablespoon pumpkin seeds
- 1 tablespoon sunflower seeds
- 1 tablespoon unsweetened dried fruit (such as raisins or cranberries)

Directions:

- In a bowl, combine all the ingredients.
- Mix well to ensure an even distribution of nuts, seeds, and dried fruit.
- Transfer the trail mix to a portable container or enjoy it immediately.

Nutritional Information:

- Calories: 220
- Total Fat: 16g
- Sodium: 0mg
- Potassium: 290mg
- Carbohydrates: 12g
- Fiber: 4g
- Sugars: 6g
- Protein: 8g

BAKED KALE CHIPS

Time: 25 minutes

Servings: 2

Ingredients:

- 4 cups kale leaves (washed, dried, and torn into bite-sized pieces)
- 1 tablespoon olive oil
- 1/4 teaspoon salt (low-sodium)

Directions:

- Preheat the oven to 325°F (165°C).

- In a large bowl, toss the kale leaves with olive oil and salt until evenly coated.

- Arrange the kale pieces in a single layer on a baking sheet.

- Bake for about 20 minutes or until the kale leaves are crispy and slightly browned.

- Remove from the oven and let them cool before serving.

Nutritional Information (per serving):

- Calories: 70
- Total Fat: 4.5g
- Sodium: 135mg
- Potassium: 310mg
- Carbohydrates: 7g
- Fiber: 2.5g
- Sugars: 0g
- Protein: 3g

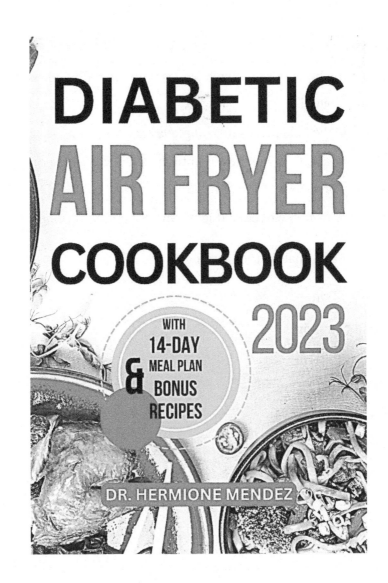

GET NOW ON AMAZON!

CHAPTER 6: DIABETIC RENAL DESSERTS

FRUIT-BASED DELIGHTS WITH REDUCED SUGAR:

BAKED CINNAMON APPLES

Time: 40 minutes

Servings: 4

Ingredients:

- 4 medium-sized apples (such as Granny Smith or Honeycrisp)
- 1 teaspoon ground cinnamon
- 1 tablespoon unsalted butter, melted
- 1 tablespoon lemon juice
- Stevia or monk fruit sweetener (optional), to taste

Directions:

- Preheat the oven to 375°F (190°C). Lightly grease a baking dish with non-stick cooking spray.

- Core the apples and cut them into thin slices. Place the apple slices in a bowl.
- In a separate small bowl, mix together the cinnamon, melted butter, and lemon juice.
- Pour the cinnamon mixture over the apple slices and toss until the apples are well coated.
- Arrange the coated apple slices in the greased baking dish in a single layer.
- Bake in the preheated oven for about 30 minutes or until the apples are tender and slightly caramelized.
- Remove from the oven and let the baked cinnamon apples cool slightly.
- Serve warm and, if desired, sprinkle with a small amount of stevia or monk fruit sweetener for added sweetness.

Nutritional Information per serving (approximately):

- Calories: 100
- Carbohydrates: 25g
- Protein: 0.5g
- Fat: 2g
- Sodium: 1mg
- Potassium: 100mg
- Phosphorus: 10mg

GRILLED PINEAPPLE WITH MINT YOGURT SAUCE

Time: 20 minutes

Servings: 4

Ingredients:

- 1 medium-sized pineapple, peeled and cored
- 1 tablespoon fresh mint leaves, chopped
- 1 cup plain Greek yogurt (low-fat or non-fat)
- 1 tablespoon lemon juice
- Stevia or monk fruit sweetener (optional), to taste

Directions:

- Preheat the grill to medium heat.
- Slice the pineapple into rings or spears.
- Place the pineapple slices on the grill and cook for about 3-4 minutes on each side until grill marks appear and the pineapple is heated through.
- Meanwhile, in a small bowl, combine the chopped mint leaves, Greek yogurt, lemon juice, and optional sweetener. Mix well.
- Remove the grilled pineapple from the heat and let it cool for a few minutes.

- Serve the grilled pineapple with a dollop of mint yogurt sauce on top.

Nutritional Information per serving (approximately):

- Calories: 80
- Carbohydrates: 16g
- Protein: 4g
- Fat: 0.5g
- Sodium: 20mg
- Potassium: 180mg
- Phosphorus: 60mg

BERRY CHIA PUDDING

Time: Overnight (plus 10 minutes of preparation)

Servings: 4

Ingredients:

- 1 cup unsweetened almond milk (or any non-dairy milk)
- 1 cup mixed berries (such as strawberries, blueberries, and raspberries), fresh or frozen
- 1/4 cup chia seeds
- 1 teaspoon vanilla extract

- Stevia or monk fruit sweetener (optional), to taste

Directions:

- In a blender, combine the almond milk, mixed berries, vanilla extract, and optional sweetener. Blend until smooth.
- Pour the berry mixture into a bowl or container with a lid.
- Add the chia seeds and stir well to combine. Make sure all the chia seeds are evenly distributed and not clumped together.
- Cover the bowl or container and refrigerate overnight or for at least 4 hours to allow the chia seeds to absorb the liquid and create a pudding-like consistency.
- Before serving, give the chia pudding a good stir to redistribute the chia seeds.
- Serve the berry chia pudding chilled and top with additional berries if desired.

Nutritional Information per serving (approximately):

- Calories: 90
- Carbohydrates: 10g
- Protein: 3g
- Fat: 5g
- Sodium: 20mg
- Potassium: 100mg
- Phosphorus: 80mg

MANGO AND COCONUT SORBET

Time: 5 minutes (plus freezing time)

Servings: 4

Ingredients:

- 2 ripe mangoes, peeled and pitted
- 1/2 cup unsweetened coconut milk
- Stevia or monk fruit sweetener (optional), to taste

Directions:

- Cut the mangoes into chunks and place them in a blender or food processor.
- Add the coconut milk to the blender.
- Blend until smooth and creamy.
- Taste the mixture and add optional sweetener if desired, blending again to combine.
- Pour the mango and coconut mixture into a shallow, freezer-safe container.
- Place the container in the freezer and let it freeze for at least 4 hours or until firm.

- Once frozen, remove the container from the freezer and let the sorbet sit at room temperature for a few minutes to soften slightly.
- Serve the mango and coconut sorbet in bowls or cones.

Nutritional Information per serving (approximately):

- Calories: 100
- Carbohydrates: 22g
- Protein: 1g
- Fat: 2g
- Sodium: 5mg
- Potassium: 200mg
- Phosphorus: 30mg

ROASTED PEACHES WITH GREEK YOGURT

Time: 30 minutes

Servings: 4

Ingredients:

- 4 ripe peaches, halved and pitted
- 1 tablespoon unsalted butter, melted
- 1 tablespoon honey (optional)

- 1 teaspoon ground cinnamon
- 1 cup plain Greek yogurt (low-fat or non-fat)

Directions:

- Preheat the oven to 375°F (190°C). Line a baking sheet with parchment paper.
- Place the peach halves, cut side up, on the prepared baking sheet.
- In a small bowl, combine the melted butter and honey (if using). Brush the mixture over the cut side of each peach half.
- Sprinkle the peaches with ground cinnamon.
- Roast the peaches in the preheated oven for about 20 minutes or until they are soft and slightly caramelized.
- Remove from the oven and let the roasted peaches cool for a few minutes.
- Serve the roasted peaches with a dollop of Greek yogurt on top.

Nutritional Information per serving (approximately):

- Calories: 120
- Carbohydrates: 20g
- Protein: 5g
- Fat: 3g
- Sodium: 30mg
- Potassium: 250mg
- Phosphorus: 60mg

DIABETIC RENAL PUDDINGS AND CUSTARDS:

VANILLA CHIA PUDDING

Time: 10 minutes (plus chilling time)

Servings: 2

Ingredients:

- 1 cup unsweetened almond milk
- 2 tablespoons chia seeds
- 1 teaspoon vanilla extract
- 1 tablespoon sugar-free sweetener (optional)
- Fresh berries or chopped nuts for topping (optional)

Directions:

- In a bowl, combine almond milk, chia seeds, vanilla extract, and sugar-free sweetener (if using). Stir well to evenly distribute the chia seeds.
- Cover the bowl and refrigerate for at least 2 hours or overnight, allowing the chia seeds to absorb the liquid and thicken the pudding.

- Once chilled and set, give the pudding a good stir to break up any clumps and achieve a smooth consistency.
- Serve the vanilla chia pudding in individual bowls or glasses. Top with fresh berries or chopped nuts, if desired.
- Enjoy this delightful and nutritious diabetic renal dessert!

Nutritional Information:

- (Per serving, without toppings)
- Calories: 80
- Total Fat: 5g
- Sodium: 40mg
- Potassium: 90mg
- Total Carbohydrates: 7g
- Fiber: 6g
- Protein: 3g

ALMOND MILK RICE PUDDING

Time: 45 minutes

Servings: 4

Ingredients:

- 1 cup cooked white rice (cooked according to package instructions)
- 2 cups unsweetened almond milk
- 2 tablespoons sugar-free sweetener
- 1 teaspoon vanilla extract
- 1/4 teaspoon ground cinnamon
- Chopped almonds or cinnamon powder for garnish (optional)

Directions:

- In a medium-sized saucepan, combine the cooked rice, almond milk, sugar-free sweetener, vanilla extract, and ground cinnamon.
- Place the saucepan over medium heat and bring the mixture to a gentle boil, stirring frequently.
- Reduce the heat to low and let the rice pudding simmer for about 30 minutes, or until the liquid is absorbed and the pudding reaches a creamy consistency.
- Remove the saucepan from heat and let the rice pudding cool slightly.
- Serve the almond milk rice pudding warm or chilled. Sprinkle chopped almonds or a dusting of cinnamon powder on top for added flavor and texture, if desired.
- Indulge in this delicious and kidney-friendly dessert!

Nutritional Information:

- (Per serving, without garnishes)
- Calories: 120
- Total Fat: 3g
- Sodium: 60mg
- Potassium: 90mg
- Total Carbohydrates: 20g
- Fiber: 1g
- Protein: 2g

COCONUT CUSTARD

Time: 1 hour 30 minutes (including chilling time)

Servings: 4

Ingredients:

- 1 can (13.5 oz) light coconut milk
- 3 large eggs
- 2 tablespoons sugar-free sweetener
- 1 teaspoon vanilla extract
- Unsweetened shredded coconut for garnish (optional)

Directions:

- Preheat the oven to 325°F (165°C).
- In a mixing bowl, whisk together the light coconut milk, eggs, sugar-free sweetener, and vanilla extract until well combined.
- Pour the custard mixture into four ramekins or oven-safe dishes.
- Place the ramekins in a baking dish and fill the dish with hot water until it reaches halfway up the sides of the ramekins.
- Carefully transfer the baking dish to the preheated oven and bake for approximately 45-50 minutes, or until the custard is set and lightly golden on top.
- Remove the baking dish from the oven and let the custard cool to room temperature.
- Once cooled, cover the ramekins with plastic wrap and refrigerate for at least 1 hour to chill thoroughly.
- Before serving, sprinkle a small amount of unsweetened shredded coconut on top for garnish, if desired.
- Savor the creamy goodness of this diabetic renal coconut custard!

Nutritional Information:

- (Per serving, without garnish)
- Calories: 140
- Total Fat: 11g
- Sodium: 35mg
- Potassium: 60mg

- Total Carbohydrates: 2g
- Fiber: 0g
- Protein: 7g

CHOCOLATE AVOCADO MOUSSE

Time: 15 minutes

Servings: 2

Ingredients:

- 1 ripe avocado, pitted and peeled
- 2 tablespoons unsweetened cocoa powder
- 2 tablespoons sugar-free sweetener
- 1/4 teaspoon vanilla extract
- 1/4 cup unsweetened almond milk
- Fresh berries for garnish (optional)

Directions:

- In a blender or food processor, combine the ripe avocado, cocoa powder, sugar-free sweetener, vanilla extract, and almond milk.
- Blend the ingredients until smooth and creamy, scraping down the sides as needed.

- Divide the chocolate avocado mousse into serving glasses or bowls.
- Refrigerate for at least 1 hour to chill and set.
- Garnish with fresh berries, if desired, before serving.
- Treat yourself to this decadent and guilt-free chocolate avocado mousse!

Nutritional Information:

- (Per serving, without garnish)
- Calories: 160
- Total Fat: 13g
- Sodium: 0mg
- Potassium: 350mg
- Total Carbohydrates: 12g
- Fiber: 8g
- Protein: 3g

LEMON PANNA COTTA

Time: 3 hours (including chilling time)

Servings: 4

Ingredients:

- 1 cup unsweetened almond milk
- 1 teaspoon unflavored gelatin
- 2 tablespoons sugar-free sweetener
- Zest of 1 lemon
- 1 tablespoon lemon juice
- Lemon slices or mint leaves for garnish (optional)

Directions:

- In a small saucepan, heat the almond milk over low heat until it is warm but not boiling.
- In a separate bowl, sprinkle the gelatin over 2 tablespoons of cold water and let it sit for a minute to soften.
- Add the softened gelatin, sugar-free sweetener, lemon zest, and lemon juice to the warm almond milk. Stir well until the gelatin is completely dissolved.
- Remove the saucepan from heat and let the mixture cool for 5-10 minutes.
- Pour the panna cotta mixture into individual ramekins or dessert cups.
- Refrigerate for at least 2 hours, or until the panna cotta is set and firm.
- Before serving, garnish with lemon slices or mint leaves for an extra touch of freshness, if desired.

- Enjoy the refreshing and tangy flavors of this diabetic renal lemon panna cotta!

Nutritional Information:

(Per serving, without garnish)

- Calories: 30
- Total Fat: 2g
- Sodium: 30mg
- Potassium: 50mg
- Total Carbohydrates: 2g
- Fiber: 0g
- Protein: 1g

INDULGENT TREATS WITH KIDNEY-FRIENDLY INGREDIENTS:

PUMPKIN SPICE MUFFINS WITH ALMOND FLOUR

Time: 40 minutes

Servings: 12 muffins

Ingredients:

- 2 cups almond flour

- 1/4 cup coconut flour
- 1 teaspoon baking powder
- 1 teaspoon baking soda
- 1/2 teaspoon cinnamon
- 1/2 teaspoon nutmeg
- 1/4 teaspoon ginger
- 1/4 teaspoon salt
- 1/2 cup pumpkin puree
- 1/4 cup unsweetened applesauce
- 3 tablespoons melted coconut oil
- 3 tablespoons honey or a sugar substitute suitable for diabetics
- 2 large eggs
- 1 teaspoon vanilla extract

Directions:

- Preheat the oven to 350°F (175°C). Line a muffin tin with paper liners or lightly grease with coconut oil.
- In a large bowl, whisk together the almond flour, coconut flour, baking powder, baking soda, cinnamon, nutmeg, ginger, and salt.
- In a separate bowl, combine the pumpkin puree, unsweetened applesauce, melted coconut oil, honey (or sugar substitute), eggs, and vanilla extract. Mix well until smooth.

- Add the wet ingredients to the dry ingredients and stir until just combined. Do not overmix.
- Divide the batter evenly among the muffin cups, filling each about 3/4 full.
- Bake for 20-25 minutes or until a toothpick inserted into the center of a muffin comes out clean.
- Remove from the oven and let the muffins cool in the tin for 5 minutes, then transfer them to a wire rack to cool completely.
- Enjoy the pumpkin spice muffins as a delicious and low-sugar treat!

Nutritional Information (per serving):

- Calories: 180
- Fat: 14g
- Carbohydrates: 10g
- Fiber: 3g
- Protein: 6g
- Sodium: 100mg
- Potassium: 130mg
- Phosphorus: 70mg

FLOURLESS CHOCOLATE CAKE

Time: 45 minutes

Servings: 8 slices

Ingredients:

- 8 ounces unsweetened baking chocolate
- 1/2 cup unsalted butter, softened
- 3/4 cup sugar substitute suitable for diabetics
- 4 large eggs
- 1 teaspoon vanilla extract
- Pinch of salt

Directions:

- Preheat the oven to 325°F (165°C). Grease a round 9-inch cake pan and line the bottom with parchment paper.
- In a microwave-safe bowl, melt the unsweetened chocolate in the microwave, stirring every 30 seconds until smooth. Set aside to cool slightly.
- In a large mixing bowl, cream together the softened butter and sugar substitute until light and fluffy.
- Add the eggs, one at a time, beating well after each addition. Stir in the vanilla extract and salt.
- Gradually add the melted chocolate to the butter mixture, mixing until well combined.

- Pour the batter into the prepared cake pan and smooth the top with a spatula.
- Bake for 30-35 minutes or until a toothpick inserted into the center of the cake comes out with a few moist crumbs.
- Allow the cake to cool in the pan for 10 minutes, then transfer it to a wire rack to cool completely.
- Serve the flourless chocolate cake as is or dust with cocoa powder for an extra touch of decadence.

Nutritional Information (per serving):

- Calories: 280
- Fat: 25g
- Carbohydrates: 11g
- Fiber: 4g
- Protein: 8g
- Sodium: 25mg
- Potassium: 200mg
- Phosphorus: 100mg

COCONUT MACAROONS (USING UNSWEETENED COCONUT)

Time: 30 minutes

Servings: 12 macaroons

Ingredients:

- 2 cups unsweetened shredded coconut
- 1/4 cup sugar substitute suitable for diabetics
- 2 large egg whites
- 1/2 teaspoon vanilla extract
- Pinch of salt

Directions:

- Preheat the oven to 325°F (165°C). Line a baking sheet with parchment paper.
- In a mixing bowl, combine the unsweetened shredded coconut and sugar substitute.
- In a separate bowl, whisk the egg whites until foamy. Add the vanilla extract and salt, and continue whisking until stiff peaks form.
- Gently fold the egg white mixture into the coconut mixture until well combined.
- Using a cookie scoop or tablespoon, drop rounded mounds of the mixture onto the prepared baking sheet, spacing them apart.
- Bake for 15-18 minutes or until the macaroons are golden brown on the edges.

- Remove from the oven and let the macaroons cool completely on the baking sheet before serving.

Nutritional Information (per serving):

- Calories: 90
- Fat: 8g
- Carbohydrates: 4g
- Fiber: 2g
- Protein: 2g
- Sodium: 30mg
- Potassium: 70mg
- Phosphorus: 30mg

PEANUT BUTTER PROTEIN BALLS

Time: 20 minutes

Servings: 12 balls

Ingredients:

- 1 cup unsalted natural peanut butter
- 1/4 cup sugar substitute suitable for diabetics
- 1/4 cup almond flour
- 1/4 cup unsweetened shredded coconut

- 2 tablespoons ground flaxseed
- 2 tablespoons unsweetened cocoa powder
- 1/2 teaspoon vanilla extract
- Pinch of salt

Directions:

- In a mixing bowl, combine the peanut butter, sugar substitute, almond flour, shredded coconut, ground flaxseed, cocoa powder, vanilla extract, and salt.
- Stir until all the ingredients are well combined and form a thick dough.
- Using your hands, roll the dough into tablespoon-sized balls.
- Place the protein balls on a parchment-lined baking sheet and refrigerate for at least 1 hour to firm up.
- Store the peanut butter protein balls in an airtight container in the refrigerator until ready to enjoy.

Nutritional Information (per serving - 1 ball):

- Calories: 150
- Fat: 12g
- Carbohydrates: 5g
- Fiber: 3g
- Protein: 6g
- Sodium: 70mg

- Potassium: 110mg
- Phosphorus: 90mg

CARROT CAKE BITES WITH CREAM CHEESE DRIZZLE

Time: 40 minutes

Servings: 12 bites

Ingredients:

- 1 cup grated carrots
- 1/2 cup almond flour
- 1/4 cup coconut flour
- 1/4 cup chopped walnuts
- 1/4 cup raisins
- 2 tablespoons sugar substitute suitable for diabetics
- 2 tablespoons melted coconut oil
- 2 tablespoons unsweetened applesauce
- 2 large eggs
- 1/2 teaspoon vanilla extract
- 1/2 teaspoon ground cinnamon
- 1/4 teaspoon ground nutmeg
- 1/4 teaspoon baking powder
- 1/4 teaspoon baking soda

- Pinch of salt

Cream Cheese Drizzle:

- 2 ounces cream cheese, softened
- 2 tablespoons sugar substitute suitable for diabetics
- 1 tablespoon unsweetened almond milk
- 1/4 teaspoon vanilla extract

Directions:

- Preheat the oven to 350°F (175°C). Line a baking sheet with parchment paper.
- In a large mixing bowl, combine the grated carrots, almond flour, coconut flour, chopped walnuts, raisins, sugar substitute, melted coconut oil, unsweetened applesauce, eggs, vanilla extract, ground cinnamon, ground nutmeg, baking powder, baking soda, and salt. Stir until well combined.
- Using a tablespoon or a cookie scoop, portion the mixture into 12 equal-sized balls. Place the balls on the prepared baking sheet and flatten slightly with the back of a spoon.
- Bake for 18-20 minutes or until the carrot cake bites are golden brown and set.
- While the bites are cooling, prepare the cream cheese drizzle. In a small bowl, whisk together the softened cream cheese, sugar

substitute, unsweetened almond milk, and vanilla extract until smooth and creamy.

- Drizzle the cream cheese mixture over the cooled carrot cake bites.
- Serve the carrot cake bites as a delightful and guilt-free treat!

Nutritional Information (per serving - 1 bite with cream cheese drizzle):

- Calories: 110
- Fat: 8g
- Carbohydrates: 7g
- Fiber: 2g
- Protein: 3g
- Sodium: 70mg
- Potassium: 110mg
- Phosphorus: 50mg

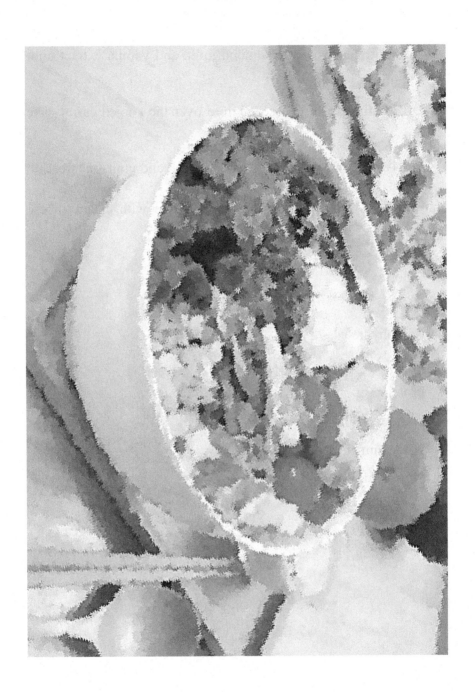

CHAPTER 7: BEVERAGES AND HYDRATION

Staying properly hydrated is essential for seniors with diabetes and kidney disease. In this chapter, we will explore a variety of refreshing and kidney-friendly beverages that can help meet your hydration needs while adhering to a diabetic renal diet. We will also provide valuable hydration tips specifically tailored to seniors, as well as offer delicious smoothie and juice recipes and suggest herbal tea blends that promote diabetic renal health. Let's dive into the world of beverages and discover delightful options to keep you hydrated and satisfied.

REFRESHING DIABETIC RENAL DRINKS:

Proper hydration is crucial for seniors with diabetes and kidney disease, as it helps maintain healthy kidney function and supports overall well-being. However, choosing the right beverages is equally important to ensure you are not consuming excess sugar, sodium, or potassium. Here are some refreshing diabetic renal drinks to quench your thirst:

157

CITRUS INFUSED WATER:

- Fill a pitcher with water and add slices of lemon, lime, and orange.
- Let it sit in the refrigerator for a few hours to allow the flavors to infuse.
- Enjoy a refreshing and hydrating drink that adds a hint of natural citrus flavor without added sugars or potassium.

CUCUMBER MINT COOLER:

- Blend fresh cucumber slices with mint leaves and water until smooth.
- Strain the mixture and pour over ice.
- Sip on this cool and hydrating beverage that also provides a refreshing taste.

HIBISCUS ICED TEA:

- Brew hibiscus tea bags in boiling water according to package instructions.
- Allow the tea to cool and pour it over ice.

Hibiscus tea is naturally caffeine-free and has been shown to have potential benefits for blood pressure management, making it a great choice for seniors with diabetes and kidney disease.

SPARKLING WATER WITH A SPLASH OF LIME:

- Fill a glass with sparkling water.
- Squeeze fresh lime juice into the glass and stir gently.
- Enjoy the effervescence and zesty flavor of this simple and hydrating beverage.

Remember to monitor your portion sizes and drink fluids in moderation, as excessive fluid intake may be harmful for individuals with compromised kidney function. It is essential to consult with your healthcare provider or a registered dietitian to determine the appropriate fluid intake for your specific health needs.

HYDRATION TIPS FOR SENIORS WITH DIABETES AND KIDNEY DISEASE:

Proper hydration is particularly important for seniors with diabetes and kidney disease, as aging can affect the body's ability to regulate fluid balance. Here are some helpful tips to stay hydrated and maintain optimal health:

MONITOR FLUID INTAKE:

- Keep track of your fluid intake throughout the day using a water bottle or a fluid intake journal.
- Aim to consume an adequate amount of fluids based on your healthcare provider's recommendations.

SPREAD FLUID INTAKE:

- Drink fluids consistently throughout the day rather than consuming a large volume at once.
- This approach can help prevent excessive fluid intake and support better hydration.

CHOOSE KIDNEY-FRIENDLY BEVERAGES:

- Opt for beverages that are low in added sugars, sodium, and potassium.
- Read labels carefully and choose options that align with your dietary restrictions and goals.

SET HYDRATION REMINDERS:

- Use timers or smartphone apps to remind yourself to drink fluids at regular intervals.
- Setting reminders can help you establish a hydration routine and prevent dehydration.

MONITOR URINE COLOR:

- Pay attention to the color of your urine, as it can indicate your hydration status.
- Pale yellow urine generally suggests good hydration, while darker urine may indicate dehydration.

BE MINDFUL OF MEDICATIONS:

- Some medications may affect fluid balance or increase the risk of dehydration.
- Consult your healthcare provider or pharmacist to understand how your medications may impact your hydration needs.

HYDRATE WITH FOODS:

- Consume hydrating foods with high water content, such as watermelon, cucumbers, oranges, and lettuce.
- These foods can contribute to your overall fluid intake and provide additional nutrients.

By incorporating these hydration tips into your daily routine and making conscious choices about your beverages, you can ensure optimal hydration and support your diabetic renal health.

KIDNEY-FRIENDLY SMOOTHIES AND JUICES:

Smoothies and juices can be a delicious way to incorporate nutrient-dense ingredients into your diet while staying hydrated. Here are some kidney-friendly smoothie and juice recipes to tantalize your taste buds:

BERRY BLAST SMOOTHIE:

- Blend a cup of mixed berries (such as strawberries, blueberries, and raspberries) with unsweetened almond milk and a handful of spinach.
- Add a scoop of protein powder for an extra nutritional boost.

GREEN POWER JUICE:

- Juice a combination of kale, celery, cucumber, and lemon for a nutrient-packed green juice.
- This juice is rich in vitamins and minerals while being low in sugar and kidney-friendly.

TROPICAL PARADISE SMOOTHIE:

- Blend frozen mango chunks, pineapple, unsweetened coconut milk, and a handful of spinach for a tropical-flavored smoothie.
- This smoothie provides a refreshing taste while offering a dose of antioxidants and fiber.

WATERMELON LIME REFRESHER:

- Blend fresh watermelon cubes with lime juice and a few mint leaves.
- This hydrating and flavorful drink is perfect for hot summer days.

Remember to adjust the recipes to accommodate your dietary needs and restrictions. You can also consult with a registered dietitian to personalize these smoothie and juice recipes based on your specific renal and diabetic requirements.

HERBAL TEA BLENDS FOR DIABETIC RENAL HEALTH:

Herbal teas can be a soothing and hydrating beverage choice for individuals with diabetes and kidney disease. Here are some herbal tea blends that can promote diabetic renal health:

DANDELION ROOT AND CINNAMON TEA:

- Combine dried dandelion root and a cinnamon stick in a teapot.
- Pour hot water over the ingredients and steep for 10-15 minutes.

Dandelion root is believed to have diuretic properties, potentially supporting kidney function, while cinnamon may help regulate blood sugar levels.

NETTLE LEAF AND GINGER TEA:

- Steep dried nettle leaves and freshly grated ginger in hot water for 5-10 minutes.

Nettle leaf is known for its potential diuretic properties, and ginger adds a warming and soothing element to the tea.

CHAMOMILE AND LAVENDER TEA:

- Combine dried chamomile flowers and dried lavender buds in a tea infuser.
- Place the infuser in a cup of hot water and steep for 5-7 minutes.

Chamomile and lavender are known for their calming properties and can contribute to relaxation and better sleep.

It is important to note that herbal teas may interact with certain medications or have specific considerations for individuals with certain health conditions. Consult with your healthcare provider before incorporating herbal teas into your routine, especially if you have any underlying medical conditions or are taking medications.

By incorporating these refreshing diabetic renal drinks, following hydration tips, enjoying kidney-friendly smoothies and juices, and savoring herbal tea blends, you can maintain optimal hydration while supporting your overall well-being.

2-WEEK DIABETIC RENAL MEAL PLAN FOR SENIORS

WEEK 1:

DAY 1:

- Breakfast: Blueberry Almond Oatmeal
- Lunch: Mediterranean Quinoa Salad
- Snack: Greek Yogurt Parfait with Berries
- Dinner: Ginger Garlic Vegetable Stir-Fry
- Dessert: Berry Chia Pudding

DAY 2:

- Breakfast: Veggie-packed Egg White Omelet
- Lunch: Grilled Lemon Pepper Cod
- Snack: Almond Butter and Apple Slices
- Dinner: Roasted Cauliflower and Brussels Sprouts
- Dessert: Vanilla Chia Pudding

DAY 3:

- Breakfast: Cinnamon Apple Oatmeal
- Lunch: Lentil and Vegetable Soup
- Snack: Celery Sticks with Hummus
- Dinner: Baked Turkey Cutlets with Steamed Broccoli
- Dessert: Almond Milk Rice Pudding

DAY 4:

- Breakfast: Coconut and Pineapple Oatmeal
- Lunch: Black Bean and Vegetable Chili
- Snack: Trail Mix with Nuts and Seeds
- Dinner: Tofu Stir-Fry with Mixed Vegetables
- Dessert: Coconut Custard

DAY 5:

- Breakfast: Peanut Butter Banana Oatmeal
- Lunch: Minestrone Soup with Kidney Beans
- Snack: Baked Kale Chips
- Dinner: Lemon Herb Salmon with Roasted Asparagus
- Dessert: Chocolate Avocado Mousse

DAY 6:

- Breakfast: Maple Pecan Oatmeal
- Lunch: Split Pea and Ham Soup (using reduced-sodium ham)
- Snack: Greek Yogurt Parfait with Berries
- Dinner: Pork Tenderloin with Sweet Potato Mash
- Dessert: Lemon Panna Cotta

DAY 7:

- Breakfast: Berry Blast Smoothie
- Lunch: Tomato Basil Soup
- Snack: Trail Mix with Nuts and Seeds
- Dinner: Szechuan Eggplant Stir-Fry
- Dessert: Mango and Coconut Sorbet

WEEK 2:

DAY 8:

- Breakfast: Kiwi and Spinach Smoothie
- Lunch: Cabbage and Carrot Clear Soup

- Snack: Almond Butter and Apple Slices
- Dinner: Grilled Chicken Breast with Herbed Quinoa
- Dessert: Roasted Peaches with Greek Yogurt

DAY 9:

- Breakfast: Blueberry Almond Oatmeal
- Lunch: Mediterranean Quinoa Salad
- Snack: Greek Yogurt Parfait with Berries
- Dinner: Ginger Garlic Vegetable Stir-Fry
- Dessert: Berry Chia Pudding

DAY 10:

- Breakfast: Veggie-packed Egg White Omelet
- Lunch: Grilled Lemon Pepper Cod
- Snack: Almond Butter and Apple Slices
- Dinner: Roasted Cauliflower and Brussels Sprouts
- Dessert: Vanilla Chia Pudding

DAY 11:

- Breakfast: Cinnamon Apple Oatmeal
- Lunch: Lentil and Vegetable Soup
- Snack: Celery Sticks with Hummus
- Dinner: Baked Turkey Cutlets with Steamed Broccoli
- Dessert: Almond Milk Rice Pudding

DAY 12:

- Breakfast: Coconut and Pineapple Oatmeal
- Lunch: Black Bean and Vegetable Chili
- Snack: Trail Mix with Nuts and Seeds
- Dinner: Tofu Stir-Fry with Mixed Vegetables
- Dessert: Coconut Custard

DAY 13:

- Breakfast: Peanut Butter Banana Oatmeal
- Lunch: Minestrone Soup with Kidney Beans
- Snack: Baked Kale Chips
- Dinner: Lemon Herb Salmon with Roasted Asparagus
- Dessert: Chocolate Avocado Mousse

DAY 14:

- Breakfast: Maple Pecan Oatmeal
- Lunch: Split Pea and Ham Soup (using reduced-sodium ham)
- Snack: Greek Yogurt Parfait with Berries
- Dinner: Pork Tenderloin with Sweet Potato Mash
- Dessert: Lemon Panna Cotta

CONCLUSION: LIFESTYLE STRATEGIES FOR OPTIMAL DIABETES AND RENAL HEALTH

In the journey of managing diabetes and renal health, it is important to not only focus on a diabetic renal diet but also adopt a holistic approach that encompasses various lifestyle strategies. In this concluding chapter, we will explore the significance of exercise and physical activity, medication management and monitoring, as well as maintaining a positive outlook and supportive network. These lifestyle strategies are vital for seniors with diabetes and kidney disease to achieve optimal health outcomes and improve their overall quality of life.

EXERCISE AND PHYSICAL ACTIVITY RECOMMENDATIONS:

Regular physical activity plays a crucial role in managing diabetes and kidney health for seniors. Engaging in exercise not only helps

173

control blood sugar levels but also contributes to weight management, cardiovascular health, and overall well-being. Before starting any exercise program, it is essential for seniors to consult with their healthcare provider, who can provide guidance based on individual needs and capabilities. Here are some exercise recommendations:

- Aerobic Exercises: Activities such as brisk walking, swimming, cycling, and low-impact aerobics are excellent choices for seniors. Aim for at least 150 minutes of moderate-intensity aerobic exercise per week, spread over several days.

- Strength Training: Including resistance exercises two to three times a week can help maintain muscle strength and improve insulin sensitivity. Use light weights, resistance bands, or bodyweight exercises to target major muscle groups.

- Flexibility and Balance Exercises: Gentle stretching and balance exercises, such as yoga or tai chi, can improve flexibility, mobility, and reduce the risk of falls.

- Stay Active Throughout the Day: Encourage regular movement throughout the day by taking breaks from sitting, performing household chores, gardening, or engaging in light physical activities.

Remember, each person has different abilities and limitations, so it's essential to tailor exercise routines to individual needs and gradually increase intensity and duration over time. Regular physical activity, even in moderate amounts, can have significant benefits for seniors with diabetes and kidney disease.

MEDICATION MANAGEMENT AND MONITORING:

Proper medication management and regular monitoring of blood glucose and kidney function are essential for seniors with diabetes and renal health issues. It is crucial to work closely with healthcare providers to develop an appropriate medication regimen and monitoring schedule. Here are some key aspects to consider:

- Medication Adherence: Follow prescribed medication instructions carefully, including dosage, timing, and potential interactions with other medications. Ensure an adequate supply of medications and discuss any concerns or side effects with healthcare providers promptly.
- Blood Glucose Monitoring: Regularly monitor blood glucose levels as recommended by healthcare providers. Use glucose meters or continuous glucose monitoring systems to track fluctuations and make informed adjustments to diet and medication if necessary.

- Kidney Function Monitoring: Seniors with kidney disease need regular monitoring of kidney function through blood tests, including serum creatinine, glomerular filtration rate (GFR), and urine albumin levels. This helps healthcare providers assess kidney health and make appropriate recommendations for diet, medication, and lifestyle adjustments.

- Collaborative Approach: Engage in open communication with healthcare providers, including doctors, nurses, dietitians, and pharmacists, to ensure coordinated care. Regularly update them on any changes in health status, medication side effects, or concerns related to diabetes or kidney health.

MAINTAINING A POSITIVE OUTLOOK AND SUPPORTIVE NETWORK:

The emotional well-being of seniors with diabetes and kidney disease is just as important as their physical health. Maintaining a positive outlook and cultivating a supportive network can significantly impact overall well-being. Here are some strategies to consider:

- Education and Empowerment: Continuously educate yourself about diabetes and kidney disease, staying informed about the latest research, treatment options, and self-care strategies. This knowledge empowers you to make informed decisions and actively participate in your health management.

- Emotional Support: Seek emotional support from family, friends, or support groups specifically for seniors with diabetes and kidney disease. Sharing experiences, challenges, and successes with others who understand can provide encouragement and motivation.

- Stress Management: Chronic stress can negatively impact blood glucose levels and overall health. Engage in stress-reducing activities such as meditation, deep breathing exercises, yoga, or hobbies that bring joy and relaxation.

- Celebrate Achievements: Recognize and celebrate small victories along the way. Acknowledge the effort and progress made in managing diabetes and kidney health, no matter how small. This positive reinforcement helps maintain motivation and a sense of accomplishment.

In conclusion, adopting a diabetic renal diet is just one aspect of managing diabetes and kidney health for seniors. Incorporating exercise and physical activity, effectively managing medications and monitoring, and maintaining a positive outlook and supportive network are equally important. By embracing these lifestyle strategies, seniors can improve their overall well-being, enhance diabetes and renal health outcomes, and enjoy a fulfilling and active life. Remember, each step taken towards better health is a step towards a brighter future.

Made in the USA
Columbia, SC
21 January 2024

30762860R00098